WHY
INDUCTION
MATTERS

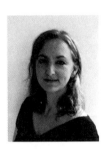

About the author

Dr Rachel Reed is a Senior Lecturer and Discipline Leader in Midwifery at the University of the Sunshine Coast, Australia. She has provided midwifery care for hundreds of women in a range of settings in the United Kingdom and Australia.

Rachel's PhD explored women's experience of birth and midwifery practice during birth. She is a writer and presenter, and is the author of the MidwifeThinking blog site. Rachel is originally from the North of England but now lives in forest in Queensland Australia.

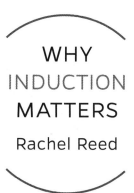

WHY
INDUCTION
MATTERS

Rachel Reed

Why Induction Matters (Pinter & Martin Why It Matters 14)

First published by Pinter & Martin Ltd 2018
reprinted 2019, 2020, 2021

©2018 Rachel Reed

ISBN 978-1-78066-600-6

Also available as an ebook

Pinter & Martin Why It Matters ISSN 2056-8657
Series editor: Susan Last
Index: Helen Bilton
Cover Design: Blok Graphic, London
Cover illustration: Sam Kalda
Proofreader: Debbie Kennett

British Library Cataloguing-in-Publication Data

A catalogue record for this book is available from the British Library.

Set in Minion

Printed and bound in the EU by Hussar

This book has been printed on paper that is sourced and harvested from sustainable forests and is FSC accredited.

Pinter & Martin Ltd
6 Effra Parade
London SW2 1PS
pinterandmartin.com

Contents

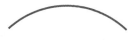

Author's Note

I gave birth to my own children before I was a midwife, and I did not have to make a decision about induction with either of my pregnancies. However, during my second pregnancy I learned that I could make choices, and that I could take ownership of those choices, and of my birth experience. After that birth I felt empowered and strong. I became a midwife because I wanted other women to know their power in childbearing, and to be supported in their decisions, whatever they may be.

As a midwife I have cared for many women having their labour induced; and many women who chose not to have their labour induced. I discovered that an empowering birth experience is not necessarily about the type of labour a woman has. It is about the woman's sense of power and her ability to make decisions about what happens to her. A woman can have an unexpected complication and emergency caesarean, yet feel empowered, respected and supported throughout.

In my role as an academic, educator and speaker I have

had the opportunity to discuss induction with a wide range of health professionals. Unfortunately, many feel poorly equipped to support women in informed decision-making, due to work pressures and a lack of confidence in their own knowledge. In practice there is a reliance on routines, norms, and guidelines that may, or may not, be evidence-based. However, there is still a great interest in this topic among health professionals, and a will to provide better support for women.

The demand for information about induction reflects the large number of women who are faced with making decisions about induction. The most popular posts on my blog MidwifeThinking are about induction. Women regularly contact me to ask questions about induction or to share their experience of induction. Often women are looking for information to help them understand what happened to them during their induction. They are seeking information they should have had before their induction took place.

I have written this book to meet the needs of women, and the health professionals who support them. The childbirth rite of passage is an opportunity for transformation and empowerment that influences a woman's sense of self and her approach to mothering. My hope is that every woman feels well informed and respected throughout her birth experience, regardless of her choices.

Introduction

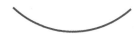

In modern maternity care systems one in four women have their labour induced.[1] Induction is a firmly established routine intervention, and many women find themselves 'booked in' to have one with little or no discussion. However, women have the right to make their own decisions about interventions recommended by health professionals. To make an informed decision about induction, women need information about why induction has been recommended, the process of induction, and the benefits and risks involved. The aim of this book is to provide comprehensive, evidence-based information, and share personal experiences about all aspects of induction. It is hoped that women will use the book as a resource to help them make their own decisions. The book is also designed to assist care providers (midwives, doulas, doctors, etc.) in sharing information with women and supporting their decisions.

Chapter 1 provides an overview of how women make decisions about induction. It describes the legal and ethical requirements of health care professionals in relation to assisting and supporting women's informed decision-making. The chapter discusses what is meant by 'evidence', and how it is used to inform maternity care guidelines and recommendations. Chapter 1 also includes a decision-making framework that can be used to evaluate your individual situation and decide what is best for you.

Chapter 2 and Chapter 3 cover the main reasons that an induction is recommended. Chapter 2 focuses on complications of pregnancy, and Chapter 3 focuses on variations of pregnancy. These chapters are large and cover many complications and variations. You can select and read the section that relates to your situation.

Chapter 4 explains how a spontaneous, physiological labour works. The content of this chapter provides the basis for understanding how induction works, and the differences between spontaneous and induced labour.

Chapter 5 and Chapter 6 explore the induction process, from preparing the body, to inducing contractions, to birthing the baby. These chapters include descriptions of the procedures used to induce labour, how they work, what they feel like, and the potential risks involved.

Chapter 7 provides an overview of common alternative methods of induction. An explanation of each approach is accompanied by an overview of research about the effectiveness of the method.

Chapter 8 is aimed at women who have decided to have their labour induced. It provides a framework for considering options, and creating a birth plan to make your induction the best possible experience for you and your baby.

Throughout this book, women share their experiences of making decisions about induction, and of the induction process. I am very grateful for their generous and honest contributions. Below the women introduce themselves:

Alice Tuson has three children. Two of her labours were induced, and her third birth she calls her 'hospital home birth'. Her three babies were born in the UK, but she now lives in Sydney, Australia and is a student midwife.

Anna Simpson is a slow cooker, having birthed her four children at home between 41 and 43 weeks' gestation. She is many things, including being a midwife, and currently lives with her husband, three daughters, one son, two dogs and her ukuleles.

Arianwen is the mother of two sons, born in different countries. She is passionate about women's rights. She enjoys coffee, laughing, and sparkling wine.

Belinda Costello is a mother of four children and an advocate for women and consumers.

Chenoa is mum to six crazy, amazing kids, three home births, and one hospital birth (triplets). She believes that our bodies CAN do this, they just need us to believe in ourselves first.

Cheree is the mother of one redheaded daughter, induced due to pre-eclampsia. Not silly enough to go back for more.

Hannah Leneham has one baby boy and had acupuncture the morning before she went into labour. She is a student nurse/midwife, and is very passionate about supporting women and their families with informed decision-making.

Hayley Murphy is mother to two young boys, and had induction experiences with both births. She is a full-time stay-at-home-mum, and part-time positive and empowering birth and breastfeeding advocate.

Hayley Jean fell pregnant with 3/4 of her nursing degree to complete. She had her son naturally via induction because of cholestasis (ICP); she then went on to complete her degree while juggling the ups and downs of motherhood. Now completed, she is expecting her second child. Hayley Jean hopes to continue studying to become a midwife.

Helen Murphy is a mother, qualified lawyer, teacher and, following her birthing experiences, now counts herself as a maternity consumer advocate.

Jade Saegenschnitter is a mother of three children, one induction resulting in an assisted vaginal birth and two spontaneous empowering births.

Jessica Offer is a master-gestator with her longest pregnancy being 44 weeks, and mother of four girls, three born at home. A writer and journalist, Jessica lives with her husband, daughters and two Burmese cats.

Jessie Johnson-Cash is a mother of two and midwife of many. She is a passionate supporter of women's choices in childbirth.

Kasia is a single mum with a teenage daughter and a newborn baby boy, studying to become a nurse.

Katrina is mother to one daughter, who entered the world surrounded by supportive midwives. Katrina is passionate about woman-centred care and choice so everyone may have a positive birth story like hers.

Kym Richter is mum to two boys, both induced, both very different births.

Kimberley Jackson is a mother of two – neither induced; one elective caesarean and one VBAC (vaginal birth after caesarean). A full-time mum, she is passionate about women knowing their options and rights so they can make an informed decision about their bodies, their births and their babies.

Lana is an environmental scientist and ocean lover. Lana has two children. The first a beautiful induction, the second at home, and she wishes that all mothers are genuinely cared for and respected.

Linda Ross is a single mother by choice to an 18-month-old who was born by induction. She just finished her first year as a part-time midwifery student while working full time, and has a strong belief in empowering women.

Lynda Hossack is a mother of six children who were all born within the hospital system, and all induced for various reasons, but mainly for post-dates (42 plus weeks). Lynda is trained as a doula but is currently growing her family. She is a self-proclaimed birth geek, and a lactivist. Her friends call her the baby/birth wikipedia.

Mariana Serra is a mother of three (an induction and two spontaneous homebirths). She became a doula after the birth of her second son.

Meg Boschetti is the mother to two beautiful girls. Her first daughter made her way into the world through induction, an experience that has taught her a lot.

Monique is a Type 1 diabetic mother of two boys, fulfilling the dream she has always held, of being at home with her children. Both her pregnancies were healthy despite her diabetes, and ended in very successful inductions and very quick labours.

Paula Dillon is a midwife, educator, wife, and mother to seven children – four in heaven and three on earth. She is passionate about childbirth and perinatal loss education, helping to break taboos around stillbirth and miscarriage, and empowering women to get to know their babies during pregnancy.

Rachel Fowler is studying to be a midwife. She has a 16-month-old son born by emergency caesarean after being induced for IUGR (intrauterine growth restriction).

Rebecca Milner is a mother of four children, none of which were induced. She is a teacher, but hopes to become a midwife in the near future.

Samantha D is a small business owner and mum to five. She has come full circle in her birthing experiences, and is dealing with birth trauma from both caesarean and vaginal births.

Samantha Hatton is a mother of one born by emergency caesarean after a breech position was discovered in labour. She is also a wife and hypnobirthing coach.

Samantha Lance is a mother of three: one heavenly baby and two rainbow babies. She has had one successful induction of labour. Samantha is a registered midwife with a special interest in pregnancy and infant loss, and caring for grieving families.

Sam Taylor is a new mum with a beautiful baby girl who was induced. She is a teacher aide and is studying towards her teacher's degree. Samantha lives with her husband and daughter.

Tessa Kowaliw has three children; her first was born via unplanned caesarean section following a failed induction, and her second two were born at home. Tessa is now an international speaker, writer and educator, using her personal experiences and skills as a consumer and advocate to consult with organisations working to measure 'what matters most', and to better understand the patient perspective.

Tiara is a mother of one boy, and is a stay-at-home mum.

Tracey Grabham is a mother of three beautiful boys (two spontaneous births and one induction). Tracey is a registered midwife.

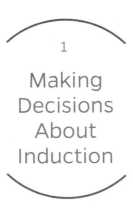

1

Making Decisions About Induction

If you are reading this book, the chances are you are looking for information to help you make a decision about induction. Making an informed decision involves considering information about your individual situation, and assessing your options. This book provides evidence-based information about induction, and shares women's experiences. It does not offer advice or recommendations about what is best for you in your individual situation. Only you can make the decision about whether to have your labour induced or not. This chapter discusses aspects of decision-making and offers a framework to assist in evaluating your options.

Roles and responsibilities in decision-making

People have the legal right to accept or decline any medical recommendation. This right even applies if declining a procedure would be life-threatening for a woman or her unborn baby. Health professionals must gain consent before carrying out any procedure, and for consent to be valid it must be voluntarily and freely given. This means that the person must not be under any undue influence or coercion, and there must be no misrepresentation about what the procedure is, or the necessity of the procedure. If these standards are not met, and a procedure is carried out without consent, that action is considered assault and battery according to law.

It is the role of health professionals to share relevant information with women to assist them in making decisions about their options in maternity care. The National Institute for Health and Care Excellence (NICE) provides guidance for health professionals about what information they should share with women when offering induction:[1]

- The reasons for induction being offered
- Where, when and how induction could be carried out
- The arrangements for support and pain relief (recognising that women are likely to find induced labour more painful than spontaneous labour)
- The alternative options if the woman chooses not to have induction of labour
- The risks and benefits of induction of labour in specific circumstances and the risks and benefits of the proposed induction methods
- That induction may not be successful and what the woman's options would be.

In addition, the health professional offering induction of labour should:

- Allow the woman time to discuss the information with her partner before coming to a decision
- Encourage the woman to look at a variety of sources of information

- Invite the woman to ask questions, and encourage her to think about her options

- Support the woman in whatever decision she makes.

The information given must be evidence-based, clearly presented, and include quantifiable numbers rather than blanket statements. For example, it is not adequate to simply state that the risk of a complication is 'increased' or 'higher' if labour is not induced. Instead, the woman must be told by how much the risk increases in comparison to waiting for spontaneous labour.

It is the responsibility of health professionals to ensure they meet the professional and legal standards relating to information-sharing. If they do this, the decision and the outcome of the decision become the responsibility of the woman. However, failing to provide adequate information, or coercing a woman into making a decision, is a breach of professional and legal standards. In these circumstances, the health professional becomes accountable for the woman's decision and any outcome related to the decision.

Research as evidence

Maternity services claim to be 'evidence-based', and this term is usually used to refer to research rather than other forms of evidence, such as experience or intuition. However, there are a number of problems with research evidence in maternity care. Routine interventions, such as induction, were introduced as part of the general medicalisation of childbirth, without any supporting research. Once routine interventions were established they became the norm within hospital practice. These practices continue today until there is good-quality research evidence to support a change. For example, until the late twentieth century women were routinely given an enema and perineal shave during labour. This only changed when research demonstrated these interventions were unnecessary and potentially harmful.

However, undertaking good-quality research into maternity care is difficult because it requires a lot of funding. Research funding is usually provided by government organisations, or the pharmaceutical and medical technology industries. Access to government funding requires research to be aligned with current health care priorities. Health care priorities tend to focus on diseases such as cancer and diabetes, rather than on maternity care. Funding by industry can alter how research is carried out, and what findings are published, because industry has a vested interest in securing a positive outcome for their product. The limitations of research funding mean that there is very little unbiased, good-quality research into induction of labour.

Where available, this book refers to Cochrane reviews when discussing research evidence. Cochrane reviews are conducted by research experts who gather every published study carried out on a topic, and assess the quality of the research and the findings. The reviews then combine the findings from all the best-quality research into one overall finding. These reviews are available online, and include a plain language summary for non-clinicians. Cochrane reviews tend to be focused on statistical findings, and provide information primarily about physical outcomes. Many of the Cochrane reviews relating to maternity care report concerns about the quantity and quality of studies. Therefore, recommendations resulting from the review are based on the limited research available.

This book also refers to clinical guidelines, primarily from (NICE) and the World Health Organisation (WHO). These guidelines are written by groups of multi-disciplinary experts, and include research evidence. However, guidelines also rely on 'expert consensus' as evidence for recommendations, and consensus tends to favour continuing a common practice rather than adopting new approaches. It can take many years for research evidence to be implemented into guidelines. Therefore, you may notice inconsistencies between research evidence and guideline recommendations in the information presented in this book.

Another important form of evidence included in this book is women's experiences of induction. There is very little research about women's experiences of induction. Therefore, I have worked with a group of women who have experience of induction to include their perspective throughout this book. As with research and guidelines, this information is not offered as advice, but as additional evidence for you to consider when making your own decisions.

Evaluating risk

The term 'risk' is used to describe a situation involving exposure to danger, or the possibility of a negative occurrence. Everything we do in life involves an element of risk, and there is no risk-free way of giving birth. International clinical guidelines suggest that induction should be offered when the danger to mother or baby if the pregnancy continues outweighs the risks of induction.[1] However, this can be difficult to determine because everyone has a different perception of risk, and there are many variables in labour and birth.

Organisations such as maternity services make evaluations of risk in a particular way. Maternity services are focused on direct organisational risk. This means minimising the risk to the organisation from legal action, increased costs of care, or reputation. The information used to evaluate risk is based on statistics about short-term, physical and measurable outcomes that impact the organisation. These statistics are generated from research about negative outcomes occurring in a general population of women, and may not be relevant for a particular woman, with her own unique health considerations. Clinical guidelines that guide health professionals' practice are based on this general type of risk assessment. Therefore, health professionals share information with women about the general, short-term, physical and measurable risks of particular options. Long-term or individual risks are usually not part of an organisation's approach to risk assessment. Health issues that arise a long time after a birth are difficult to clearly link back to the care provided during birth. In addition, emotional and psychological outcomes are difficult to measure, and are unlikely to impact the organisation. For example, a woman who is experiencing depression or psychological trauma due to her birth experience will access support through her general practitioner and mental health services, rather than from maternity services. Therefore, the cost of this care is not a risk to the organisation where she gave birth.

In maternity services the threshold for intervening to reduce a particular risk is very low if the impact of the possible outcome is considered very significant. For example, induction of labour for post-dates pregnancies is based on a less than 0.3% chance of stillbirth if a pregnancy continues beyond 41 weeks (see chapter 3). While 0.3% is a small number, the impact of stillbirth is extremely high for the families who experience it. Comparing this one particular risk with the risks of induction can be very complex. Induction involves a number of risks, including, for example, postpartum haemorrhage (see chapter 6), that are much more likely to occur than a 0.3% chance of stillbirth. In addition, other risks of induction, such as a caesarean, carry additional long-term and short-term risks for mother and baby.

The only person who can effectively assess the risk of anything is the person who will be affected by the outcome. Therefore, it is up to the woman who has been offered an induction to evaluate risks in her own individual situation, and choose the right option for her. It can be helpful to consider the general statistical risks associated with inducing and not inducing. However, it is also important to consider other risks that are important to the individual, for example, the experience of birth, and emotional and psychological factors.

How decisions are made

Decisions are not based purely on rational and objective information. Emotions and feelings drive decision-making, and social and cultural norms influence emotions and feelings.[2] Following the recommendations of health professionals is a social norm, and there is a cultural perception that health professionals are experts who know what is best for individuals. Our culture tends to prefer the scientific information that health professionals share over the personal knowledge of an individual woman. Therefore, the vast majority of women decide to follow health professionals' recommendations, particularly with their first baby. Making decisions against social and cultural norms can be emotionally challenging, and women are socialised into being compliant with authority figures rather than to ask questions and assert their wishes.

However, on an individual level, decisions are influenced by more than just social and cultural norms. Personal experience is one of the most influential factors in decision-making. A woman who has previously had an induction may feel more or less positive about choosing this option again based on her experience. Individual women are also strongly influenced by the experiences and advice of their family and friends.

Decision-making is not as simple as looking at statistics and making a choice based on the best number. Pre-existing beliefs and opinions influence how we seek and interpret information. When making a decision we tend to start with a preference for one option, then seek information to support that option. The internet has made this approach even easier because it has increased our access to information, and to people who will reinforce our beliefs and choices. This is not necessarily an incorrect way to make a decision about induction; choosing an option that is aligned with personal beliefs is how we make most decisions in life. However, it is important to understand that personal biases might alter decision-making in relation to induction.

I didn't believe I had a choice with my first daughter when I was induced with her in hospital. I felt like I had no rights. With my second, third and fourth daughters I decided not to be induced because of my previous experience. I researched actual statistics, learned about birth and hormones and followed my intuition. I trusted in my midwives, but also didn't feel afraid to ask questions or decline choices based on my own belief or vibe. Jessica

When I was looking at getting induced with my daughter I spoke to my midwife who recommended me not to go through with it as she reckoned my baby wasn't as big as the ultrasound was stating. I read all the brochures she gave me, my partner got online and researched different things. I also spoke to a very close friend who got induced with her first as I knew she would tell me the good and the bad of all of it, and give me her honest opinion about the whole thing. We wanted to make sure we looked at it from all angles because we knew once we started we weren't going to turn back. We were always leaning towards getting induced and after all the pros and cons and listening to all the stories I was still all for getting induced. Sam

With my first baby, I didn't think I had a choice and was happy to just do as I was told. I trusted their advice and just let things happen. With my third baby I did lots of reading of evidence-based information on gestational diabetes and induction. I spoke a lot with my Midwifery Group Practice midwife and student midwife, as well as with peers and online groups geared towards natural birthing. I decided there wasn't enough evidence to warrant an induction for my situation. I knew a lot more and knew it was my choice. Jade

I used the following in my decision-making: my readings about normal birth, birth physiology and hormones, and the cascade of interventions. I used my intuition about my body and baby, and my awareness (or lack thereof) of my rights and options. For later births, my knowledge of the hospital policies and guidelines helped. I used a particular website fairly extensively, including the references provided and the internet rabbit holes they led me down. I used the advice of my midwives, and the awareness of my own social supports. And I used my own beliefs about what I did and didn't want my body to experience, and how I felt about being touched. Anna

After my 36-week scan, it was recommended I have an induction at 38 weeks [for growth restriction]. *I was not pressured. In fact I was supported. My obstetrician and midwife did not push me, they simply presented me with the facts, the options and the recommendations. I further did my own research and agreed for an induction. I was given options on the process, and fully supported.* Tracey

My induction was a train wreck, ending in an emergency caesarean. The most powerful factor in my decision-making process was misinformation given to me by obstetricians because unfortunately, despite my prior reading, as a first-time mum I just didn't understand the reality that in a hospital system, often you are told what you need to hear to make a decision that's convenient for them. Baby number two was a polar opposite experience. I knew that I would never again agree to an induction. Leading up to the birth, I let my intuition guide my choices.　　　　　　　　*Helen*

For my fifth babe I was seeing community midwives for a period, and at every appointment a different midwife would tell me different policies for the same birth location. Once I enlisted my 1–1 midwife, we explored all options with reference to research studies, personal experiences, and professional advice.　　　　　　　　*Samantha D*

For my first baby I expected I'd go over my due date. I tried every home remedy under the sun (or at least available on Google, which is A LOT). I let the hospital book me in to be induced 12 days post-dates because I was told they had to. I did some really bad (Google) research on the induction process because the hospital was vague, and I didn't know what to ask. And I allowed a few people to get inside my pregnant head about how bad it would be for my baby to be born on Christmas Day (in hindsight I see how stupid that concern was, but in the moment it felt like an important detail). I had no idea what I was getting myself into, or how it would affect me psychologically after. I had family coaching me about informed consent, and reminding me that they couldn't make me do anything, but in my world it was the done thing when you go well past your due date so it shouldn't have been a big deal, right? Oh so wrong!　　　*Meg*

A decision-making framework

The following framework is for those who like a systematic approach to decision-making. The framework will guide you through the process of considering information and reflecting on your thoughts about your situation and options. You might like to write notes in response to the questions posed, and discuss your thoughts with your family, friends and care provider.

1. Consider the reason that induction has been offered
Induction is offered when there is a concern for the wellbeing of the mother or baby if the pregnancy continues. It is important to understand why induction has been recommended, and what the potential complications are if you decline induction. Read the section in 'complications of pregnancy' (chapter 2) or 'variations of pregnancy' (chapter 3) relevant to your situation and consider the following questions:

a) Is your situation a complication or a variation?
A complication is a condition such as pre-eclampsia, where there is already a problem occurring. A variation is a situation where mother and baby are currently well, but the variation may increase the chance of a complication occurring in the future.

b) What are the complications associated with your situation?
Why has an induction been offered? What are the general chances of these complications occurring? Do you have any individual factors that may alter the chance of a complication occurring for you? Are you or your baby currently showing signs of a complication occurring now? Are there immediate concerns for you or your baby's health?

c) Will inducing your labour reduce the chance of these complications occurring?

How will induction reduce the chance of a complication? How much will induction reduce the chance of a complication occurring in comparison to not inducing?

2. Consider the experience of induction

An induced labour is very different from a spontaneous labour, and it is important to understand the differences and how they might alter your expectations and experience of labour. First read chapter 4 about spontaneous labour to gain an understanding of physiological labour and birth. Then read chapters 5 and 6 about the induction process and chapter 7 about alternative methods of induction. Consider the following questions:

a) *What were your thoughts about labour before an induction was offered?*
Did you have particular expectations or preferences about your labour?

b) *How will the induction process alter your previous expectations about your labour?*
How will your plans for labour change if you are induced? For example, will you need to re-consider your choices about pain relief, or your place of birth?

c) *What are the risks of induction in your situation?*
What are the general risks of induction? Do you have factors that will increase or decrease the general risks of induction? For example, will this be your first labour, or have you experienced labour before? Does your complication or variation alter the risks of induction (see the relevant section in chapter 2 or 3)?

d) *What are your thoughts about alternative methods of induction?*
Are there any alternative methods of induction that you would consider using? What are the risks and benefits of

those alternative methods in your situation? Would you use these methods instead of, or in addition to medical induction?

3. Consider the alternative options to induction

Waiting for spontaneous labour
Consider the following questions about waiting for spontaneous labour:

a) *What are the risks of waiting for spontaneous labour?*
   See your answer to question 1b. Are there additional individual risks you can identify? For example, a family member being unavailable to support you after a certain date.

b) *Is there anything you can do to reduce these risks?*
   Are there any changes you can make to reduce the chance of a complication occurring? For example, keeping your blood sugars within a normal range if you have been diagnosed with gestational diabetes (see chapter 2).

c) *Will additional monitoring help to identify a complication early?*
   What monitoring is offered in your situation? Will this monitoring identify a complication early enough to manage it? Often additional monitoring of you and your baby will be recommended if you choose to wait. However, in most cases this monitoring does not improve outcomes. Refer to the relevant section in chapter 2 or 3 for information about additional monitoring in your situation.

d) *How do you feel about additional monitoring?*
   Will monitoring reassure you, or make you more worried and stressed?

e) *What are your boundaries and thresholds about waiting?*

Will you re-evaluate your decision and options at a particular point? For example, if the pregnancy reaches a particular gestation, or if your situation changes and a variation becomes a complication.

f)   *What support will you have from family and friends while you wait?*
Will your family and friends support your decision to wait? If not, how will you minimise any stress caused by the lack of support, and gain support elsewhere?

Planned caesarean

In some circumstances a planned caesarean may be an alternative option to induction. However, caesarean surgery carries a number of short-term and long-term risks, for the mother and baby, and increases the chance of complications in future pregnancies (see page 69).[3] In addition, some conditions, such as pre-eclampsia and gestational diabetes, increase the chance of complications occurring during and after surgery. If your care provider has offered an induction rather than a planned caesarean, it suggests that the risks of a caesarean are higher than those of an induction in your situation. However, in some circumstances, such as a severely growth-restricted baby (see page 47), the risks of induction may be higher, and a planned caesarean might be a better option. You will need to discuss the specifics of your situation, and the option of a caesarean, with your care provider.

4. Make your decision

Evaluate the information you have considered in the previous questions. Create a summary for yourself using the BRAIN framework – Benefits, Risks, Alternatives, Intuition, Now/ Nothing:[4]

BENEFITS	What are the benefits of induction for you? This may include non-physical benefits, such as not having to worry about a complication occurring if the pregnancy continues.
RISKS	What are the risks of induction for you? This may include how induction will alter your wishes for your labour experience.
ALTERNATIVES	What are your alternative options?
INTUITION	What is your intuition or gut feeling telling you?
NOW/NOTHING	The 'N' in BRAIN can be used to consider 'now' and 'nothing'. Does this decision need to be made now? Is there urgency about your situation? What would happen if you did nothing? If you choose to do nothing, when do you want to re-evaluate your options?

5. Communicate your decision

Once you have made your decision you will need to share it with your care provider. This can be the most challenging aspect of making a decision, particularly when you are choosing to decline a medical recommendation. However, it is your care provider's professional obligation to respect and support your decision. They will be required to document that you have declined their recommendation, and record that they provided you with information about the risks involved.

If your care provider does not respect your decision, you have the right to ask to see an alternative care provider and/or the person in charge of maternity services. You can also access support through consumer organisations (see additional resources page 154).

While health professionals must provide evidence to support their recommendations, you are not obligated to provide evidence to support your decision, or discuss your reasons why. You are entitled to make a decision that is not aligned with recommendations, or your care provider's preferences. Ultimately you are responsible for how you make your decision and the outcome of your decision.

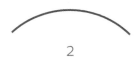

2

Complications
of Pregnancy

Complications of pregnancy are health problems that occur during pregnancy. In some cases the health problem is directly caused by the pregnancy and will resolve once the baby is born. In other cases, a pre-existing health problem is worsened by pregnancy. Induction of labour is recommended for some complications when it is considered that the wellbeing of mother and/or baby is in danger if the pregnancy continues. This chapter discusses the main complications of pregnancy which lead to a recommendation to induce labour. Research, guidelines, and women's experiences are discussed to help readers make their own decisions about induction.

High blood pressure

High blood pressure (hypertension) is a common complication of pregnancy. Blood pressure is measured by taking two recordings, for example 120/70mmHg (mmHg means millimetres of mercury). The first recording represents 'systolic' pressure, which reflects the pressure of blood being pumped out of the contracting heart muscle. The systolic blood pressure varies when the heart pumps harder, for example during exertion or stress. The second recording represents 'diastolic' pressure, which reflects the pressure of blood when the heart relaxes between contractions. The diastolic pressure is dependent on the health of blood vessels throughout the body. Healthy blood vessels stretch in response to the pressure of blood leaving the heart, slowing down the force of blood as it circulates. Therefore, diastolic blood pressure is lower than systolic blood pressure. Unhealthy blood vessels are less flexible and remain narrow as blood flows through them, causing the pressure of the blood to remain high. You can see this effect on water flowing through a hosepipe. If you compress the hose to make the pipe narrower, the water pressure increases. The standard definition of high blood pressure is a systolic of 140mmHg or more, and/or a diastolic of 90mmHg or more.

Blood pressure normally changes during pregnancy due to the influence of pregnancy hormones and increased blood volume. Early in pregnancy progesterone acts on the blood vessels to soften them, resulting in a lowering of blood pressure from around 12 weeks. It is helpful to have a blood pressure measurement taken before this occurs, so you have an accurate baseline from which to assess any rise in blood pressure later in pregnancy. The baby grows significantly between 24 and 36 weeks, and the mother's blood volume increases by nearly 50% to support this growth. Her heart needs to pump harder to circulate the additional blood, making the pressure of the blood coming out of the heart higher. This higher blood pressure balances out the blood pressure lowering effect of softer blood vessels, bringing the blood pressure back to pre-pregnant levels or a little higher. High blood pressure in pregnancy is defined using the same normal range as for non-pregnant people (see above). However, in addition, a rise of 30mmHg over a woman's pre-pregnancy blood pressure is considered to be abnormally high for that individual woman. For example, if a woman had a pre-pregnancy blood pressure of 100/60 mmHg, then a change of blood pressure to 130/90 mmHg would be of concern.

High blood pressure can occur during pregnancy in the absence of any other problems. Some women already have high blood pressure (chronic hypertension) before they become pregnant, and this may not be identified until they have their blood pressure taken during routine antenatal care. Other women will develop high blood pressure in response to changes in pregnancy. This is called 'pregnancy-induced hypertension' (PIH). Most women with high blood pressure in pregnancy have an otherwise healthy pregnancy. However, high blood pressure does increase the chance of other complications occurring, such as pre-eclampsia, pre-term birth and problems with the function of the placenta (see growth-restricted baby). Medication may be recommended to lower blood pressure to reduce the chance of these complications.[1]

There are two approaches to induction of labour for high blood pressure in the absence of additional complications. The first is to induce labour before any complications occur. However, most women with high blood pressure do not go on to develop complications. Induction also does not improve outcomes for the baby if their mother has high blood pressure.[2] The second approach is to wait for spontaneous labour unless blood pressure worsens or other complications arise. NICE recommends that for women whose blood pressure is lower than 160/110mmHg, the timing of birth should be discussed with an obstetrician, taking into account the whole clinical picture.[1]

I had high blood pressure from about 28 weeks. Not high enough to be medicated, but high enough that my midwife was concerned. She didn't want me birthing at home past 41 weeks because of my high blood pressure. So at 40+3 weeks I consented to a stretch and sweep. I went into labour the following night. Long story short, I ended up with a caesarean after lots of nipple stimulation, clary sage oil and an ARM [artificial rupture of membranes]. Labour didn't progress past 4cm dilated. In hindsight I wonder how different things would have been had I declined that stretch and sweep. I see it as the first in a cascade of interventions. I wasn't worried about the health of me or my baby (I knew we were okay), but I didn't want to lose the chance to birth at home. Jessie

Pre-eclampsia

Pre-eclampsia begins early in pregnancy when the blood vessels in the placenta implant into the uterus abnormally, reducing blood flow to the placenta and baby. The mother's body responds by releasing substances that act on the blood vessels throughout her body. The blood vessels tighten and constrict repeatedly, which increases blood pressure. Over time, the walls of the blood vessels become damaged and develop small holes that allow fluid to leak out into the tissues causing oedema (fluid retention). Protein is released into the bloodstream to fix these holes, but it also leaks out of the blood vessels. When protein leaks out of the blood vessels in the kidneys it ends up being excreted in urine (proteinuria). The three most common symptoms of pre-eclampsia are high blood pressure, oedema and protein in the urine. If pre-eclampsia progresses it can cause problems throughout the body resulting in additional symptoms including headaches, visual disturbances and pain in the liver (upper right area of the abdomen). Even though pre-eclampsia begins in early pregnancy, the symptoms do not usually appear until after 20 weeks, commonly becoming apparent towards the end of pregnancy. Routine antenatal assessments of blood pressure and urine dipsticks can identify symptoms of pre-eclampsia. However, the diagnosis of pre-eclampsia is made based on the results of a blood test that assesses whether organs such as the liver and kidneys are functioning normally.

The complications caused by pre-eclampsia are significant for both mother and baby. If left untreated the woman can experience kidney and liver failure, bleeding in the brain, eclampsia (seizures), and problems with blood clotting. Because the placenta has reduced blood flow, the baby can become growth restricted and/or be born prematurely. The risks of pre-eclampsia can be minimised with medications; however, the only cure is the birth of the baby and the placenta. Therefore, induction of labour is recommended in the case of pre-eclampsia.[1] The ideal timing for induction will depend on how severe the pre-eclampsia and symptoms are. Usually induction is offered after 37 weeks to reduce the risks of pre-term birth. However, if the mother or baby are very unwell, induction may be recommended earlier.

An induction for pre-eclampsia usually involves additional interventions such as medication to lower blood pressure and reduce the risk of seizure. An epidural may also be recommended because the anaesthetic used in an epidural relaxes blood vessels and reduces blood pressure. Even when mother and baby are unwell a caesarean will be avoided if possible, because pre-eclampsia alters blood clotting and increases the chance of surgical complications.

With my first and only pregnancy and birth, I was planning a home birth until pre-eclampsia came along at about 32 weeks. At about 36+4 weeks, my blood pressure was slightly more elevated than normal and I think my bloods were abnormal. I was told to stay in hospital overnight for blood pressure monitoring, so my husband and sister went home. At 1am a registrar came in all loaded up, and stated they had decided to induce me with gel. I asked for a few minutes to think about it all, as I was only aware I was in for monitoring. I tried calling my husband and sister, but both were asleep. I'd had a crap pregnancy so quite frankly I was happy to get her out. In hindsight, I think we were both very lucky she came out at 36+4/5, on the small side, 2.5kg [5lb 5oz], but no need for any interventions. I on the other hand had a retained placenta, lost 2.5 litres of blood and had a 2nd degree tear so ended up in theatre.   *Cheree*

Diabetes

Diabetes occurs when the body is unable to either produce enough insulin, or respond normally to insulin. Insulin is secreted by beta cells in the pancreas, and is required by cells in the body to convert glucose (carbohydrates) from the diet into energy. Without normal insulin, glucose in the blood remains unconverted, resulting in abnormally high blood glucose levels. Healthy blood glucose levels for non-pregnant people are 4.0 to 6.0 mmol/L (millimoles per litre) when fasting, and up to 7.8 mmol/L two hours after eating.

Gestational diabetes

The term 'gestational diabetes' refers to diabetes that is first diagnosed during pregnancy. The vast majority of women with gestational diabetes have what is called 'pregnancy-induced diabetes'. However, a small percentage of women diagnosed with gestational diabetes have undetected 'pre-existing diabetes' (see below) that they only find out about through antenatal testing. It is not possible to know whether a woman has pregnancy-induced diabetes, or pre-existing diabetes, until after her pregnancy ends. After the baby is born, blood glucose levels return to normal if the diabetes was pregnancy induced. Therefore, any diabetes identified during pregnancy is treated as gestational diabetes.

Pregnancy changes the way the body responds to insulin. The placenta produces hormones that support the baby's growth and development. From 20 weeks' gestation these hormones cause insulin resistance in the mother's cells. Cells that are resistant to insulin are less able to convert glucose into energy. However, the pancreas increases production of insulin during pregnancy to compensate for insulin resistance. This additional insulin keeps blood glucose levels within a normal range. In gestational diabetes the pancreas is unable to secrete enough additional insulin to maintain normal blood glucose.

There is disagreement about the best approach to screening and diagnosis of gestational diabetes. In the United Kingdom, NICE warns that over-diagnosis of gestational diabetes leads to increased antenatal monitoring, and increased interventions during labour, without significantly improving outcomes.[3] Therefore, in the United Kingdom screening is offered only to women with known risk factors for developing gestational diabetes. In contrast, Australia and the United States offer routine screening to all pregnant women. The standard test for gestational diabetes is the 'oral glucose tolerance test' (OGTT), where a blood sample is taken before and two hours after drinking a glucose solution. However, there is disagreement about what level of blood glucose should be used to diagnose gestational diabetes. In recent years the range of what is defined as 'normal' blood glucose levels has been lowered, resulting in many more women being diagnosed as diabetic, particularly in countries with routine screening. For example, the incidence of gestational diabetes varies from 3% to 18% of pregnancies, depending on the definition used, the approach to screening, and the population of women.[4]

Determining risk in gestational diabetes is complicated. The research into gestational diabetes does not distinguish between women with pre-existing diabetes, and those with pregnancy-induced diabetes. In addition, research often combines the outcomes for women who were able to maintain normal blood glucose levels and those who did not. What is known is that the complications associated with gestational diabetes are to do with blood glucose levels, not the diagnosis, or type of diabetes. The treatment of gestational diabetes aims to keep blood glucose within normal limits either by diet and lifestyle changes or, in some cases, by medication. If a woman with gestational diabetes keeps her blood glucose within normal limits, her chance of complications is the same as a woman who does not have diabetes.

For women, abnormally high blood glucose levels in pregnancy increase the chance of a number of complications, including pre-eclampsia, excess amniotic fluid, postpartum haemorrhage and infection. In addition, a woman who has gestational diabetes is more likely to develop type 2 diabetes and cardiovascular disease later in life. Gestational diabetes can also affect the baby during pregnancy, as the mother's high blood glucose crosses the placenta into the baby's blood circulation. In response, the baby increases their own insulin production to clear the additional blood glucose. High levels of insulin in the baby's body stimulate the growth of organs, and result in additional fat storage around the abdomen and shoulders. Larger shoulders can increase the chance of the baby having difficulty getting through the pelvis during birth (see page 71).

Once the baby is born, she or he will need to readjust their insulin production to deal with the withdrawal of their mother's high blood glucose. It is very common for the baby's own blood glucose levels to drop too low (hypoglycaemia) while this adjustment takes place. Babies are often given formula milk to increase their blood glucose levels, which can disrupt their gut microbiome and interfere with establishing breastfeeding.[5] Colostrum (first breastmilk) has very high levels of glucose and can help to stabilise the baby's blood glucose without the risks of formula. Women can express colostrum after 36 weeks of pregnancy so that they have an additional supply of colostrum in case their baby needs it during the first days of life.[6] The baby also needs to break down and excrete the additional red blood cells that they made in response to insulin. It is common for babies to develop jaundice during this process, because the by-product of breaking down red blood cells is bilirubin, a yellow substance. Excess bilirubin causes the yellowing of the baby's skin and eyes that is referred to as jaundice. In some cases, light therapy is needed to help to break down the bilirubin and disperse it back into the baby's circulation, where it is processed by the liver and excreted out in the baby's urine and stool. Additional colostrum and breastmilk can increase the amount of urine and stools the baby passes, helping them to excrete the bilirubin quicker.

Less common complications for babies subjected to high blood glucose include premature birth and respiratory distress syndrome. However, these complications may be associated with early induction for diabetes causing pre-term birth. Long-term risks include the development of obesity and type 2 diabetes later in life. Some studies have suggested there is an increased risk of stillbirth for women with gestational diabetes.[7] However, a recent Cochrane review found no stillbirths among a group of 425 women with gestational diabetes.[8]

The Cochrane review also concluded that there is insufficient evidence to demonstrate differences in outcomes for women with gestational diabetes and their babies if they have their labour induced or wait for spontaneous labour.[8] The poor quantity and quality of research about gestational diabetes has led to varying recommendations about induction. For example, NICE (United Kingdom) recommends that women with gestational diabetes should be advised to give birth before 41 weeks gestation, and be offered an induction to achieve this.[3] In contrast, the World Health Organization recommends that induction of labour should not be offered for gestational diabetes unless there is evidence of other abnormalities occurring, such as abnormal blood glucose levels.[9] Australian guidelines also state that if blood glucose is well managed, there is no indication for induction for gestational diabetes.[10]

I had gestational diabetes with my 3rd pregnancy. My midwife had spoken at length with me about what the hospital would suggest to me, and that ultimately it was my choice. I was put on metformin [medication to help regulate blood glucose] *for my fasting levels, I didn't want to take it but felt I should. My baby was growing perfectly. At my 37-week appointment the obstetric consultant said 'OK we will book your induction for 38–39 weeks'. I told her 'No, I won't be having an induction.' I explained that I didn't feel it was best for me or my baby. The obstetrician tried to change my mind by mentioning a few times that babies can just die. She then told me I should have a stretch and sweep instead, and she wanted it done that week. I said from 38 weeks I would consider it. At my next appointment the obstetrician mentioned they like to induce women on metformin at 38 weeks, but could see that I'd declined (in my notes). She spoke about why they suggest it, and I said I understood but didn't feel it was the right choice for me yet. She understood and respected my decision. My midwife and I then had an appointment and discussed induction. She fully supported me to say no. I had a stretch and sweep at 38+2 weeks because I was a little bit worried despite all my research. In hindsight I wouldn't have done that. My baby was born the next evening.* Jade

Pre-existing diabetes

Pre-existing diabetes is diagnosed before pregnancy begins. There are two types of diabetes, type 1 and type 2. Type 1 diabetes is caused by an autoimmune condition in which the insulin-producing cells in the pancreas are destroyed. The pancreas can no longer produce insulin, and insulin medication is needed to maintain normal blood glucose levels. This type of diabetes is commonly diagnosed in childhood or early adulthood. Type 2 diabetes occurs when the body becomes resistant to the normal effects of insulin, or loses the capacity to produce enough insulin. Type 2 diabetes is progressive, and usually starts later in life.

The risks associated with pre-existing diabetes include those for abnormal blood glucose levels in gestational diabetes (see above). However, because the baby can be subjected to high blood glucose from the beginning of pregnancy, rather than from 20 weeks, there are additional risks, including an increased chance of miscarriage, stillbirth and congenital abnormality. Well-managed blood glucose levels reduce the chance of complications considerably. In recent years the stillbirth rate for women with type 1 and type 2 diabetes has significantly reduced due to improvements in the management of blood glucose in pregnancy.[11] However, in the case of pre-existing diabetes this does not eliminate the risks in the same way as for pregnancy-induced diabetes. In particular, there remains an increased chance of complications for women with type 1 diabetes. Due to this, guidelines usually recommend offering induction before 39 weeks' gestation for both types of pre-existing diabetes.[3]

I was diagnosed with type 1 diabetes at the age of 25. Once I was pregnant at age 26, I discussed labour and birth with my obstetrician and endocrinologist. It was highly recommended that I undergo an induction of labor. I was told that, although my blood sugar levels were extremely well controlled and no complications had arisen, by simply having type 1 diabetes the risks associated with going to full term outweighed the risks associated with an early labour. My obstetrician explained that not everything about type 1 diabetes and pregnancy was yet known, and it would be better to be on the safe side. I agreed. I choose to follow my doctor's advice as I believed controlling my labour and monitoring my baby would put me more at ease than not knowing, and not having control. I did feel that the induction was most likely unnecessary in my situation, as do a number of other women with type 1 diabetes I have met. But as my doctor explained, we do it not because of what we do know, or what has happened, but because of what we don't, and what could happen. My induction was successful, my labour was only four hours, I tolerated the pain fine, and my baby did not need any time in special care. Monique

Intrahepatic cholestasis of pregnancy

Intrahepatic cholestasis of pregnancy (ICP) is also referred to as obstetric cholestasis. This disorder involves a slowing down, or interruption, of bile flow (cholestasis) that begins in the liver (intrahepatic), and occurs only during pregnancy, resolving after the baby is born. ICP results in a build-up of bile acids in the liver, which then leak out into the bloodstream.

The cause of ICP is unclear, but it may be due to a combination of hormonal, genetic, and environmental factors.

The main symptom of ICP is itching (pruritus), usually occurring after 28 weeks' gestation, although it can begin earlier in pregnancy. Itching tends to be focused on the hands and feet, but can be anywhere on the body. Itching can be constant or intermittent, and is often worse at night, causing disturbed sleep. Women can find the itching very distressing and uncomfortable, and while there is no rash with ICP, women often mark their own skin from scratching. Other symptoms include dark urine, pale stools, pain around the liver (upper right side of the abdomen), loss of appetite, exhaustion and feeling generally unwell. Less commonly, ICP causes yellowing of the skin and eyes (jaundice).

Testing for ICP is only offered to women who report symptoms, or who have a history of ICP. Blood samples are taken, and bile acid levels and liver function are assessed. Raised bile acid levels are used to diagnose ICP. However, the levels considered 'abnormal' can be inconsistent across laboratory testing techniques, health facilities and guidelines. The ICP Support Organisation, a research-based charity, suggests that a standardised reference is needed to avoid confusion, and that bile acid levels over 14μmol/L should be classified as abnormal.[12] A liver function test assesses a number of enzymes in the blood to assess how well the liver is functioning. However, a diagnosis of ICP is based on bile acid levels only, so abnormal liver function is not considered ICP unless bile acids are also abnormal. If the results of either test are normal but symptoms persist, it is important to repeat the blood tests. Some women experience symptoms for weeks before their blood tests become abnormal.

ICP is uncommon, affecting less than 1% of pregnant women in the United Kingdom.[13] Therefore, there is limited research available that assesses the risks of the condition. Women with gestational diabetes, pre-eclampsia and twin pregnancies are more likely to develop ICP.[14] This overlap of conditions makes research specifically looking at ICP more difficult. Most women follow recommendations for early induction, so there are no studies looking at women who progress beyond 38 weeks' gestation with ICP. The research that is available identifies a number of risks associated with ICP.[12] For the woman, the main risks of ICP are associated with severe itching: for example, damage to the skin from scratching, and psychological stress due to lack of sleep. Symptoms of ICP usually resolve within a few weeks after the baby is born. However, some women will continue to experience hormone-related itching, for example during particular times in their menstrual cycle, or with the contraceptive pill. Women with ICP can also experience gallstones before, during, or after their pregnancy, and are at increased risk of developing type 2 diabetes and/or cardiovascular disease later in life. The recurrence risk of ICP in subsequent pregnancies is around 60-90%.[12]

The risks of ICP for the baby appear to be linked to bile acid levels, and the higher the levels, the greater the chance of a complication occurring. Exactly how increased bile acids cause complications is still largely unknown, and difficult to determine. For example, bile acids may act on uterine muscle, causing contractions, and in some cases pre-term labour, and the rate of pre-term labour is higher for women with ICP (25% compared to 6.5%).[15] However, this includes babies who were induced before 37 weeks, as well as those born spontaneously before 37 weeks. Considering that many women have their pregnancies induced early due to ICP, the rate of spontaneous pre-term labour is difficult to establish. Babies born to women with ICP are more likely to have passed meconium (see pages

64–66), even if they are pre-term. This is not linked to distress, and may be due to increased movement of fluids through the bowel caused by bile acids. Babies are also more likely to need additional support immediately after birth to establish breathing, and this may be due to the effects of bile acids on the surfactant in the lungs. Surfactant is a substance that helps the baby's lungs to inflate and stay open after birth. As a result of initial breathing problems and/or pre-term birth, ICP babies are more likely to be admitted to a special care unit after birth (12% compared to 5.6% of non-ICP babies).[15] However, admission is usually short term and babies of ICP mothers tend to recover well.

The most concerning risk associated with ICP is stillbirth. The rate of stillbirth is higher than in non-ICP pregnancies, and varies with gestational age.[16] For example, at 36 weeks' gestation there is a general stillbirth rate of 0.06% compared to 0.02% for non-ICP pregnancies; and at 40 weeks there is a stillbirth rate of 0.2% compared to 0.06%. The cause of ICP-related stillbirth is still under investigation, but it may be linked to bile acids. Stillbirth rates are higher for women with bile acid levels over 40μmol/L, and increase as the bile acid levels rise. However, studies have also demonstrated the unpredictable nature of ICP after 36 weeks. For example, some babies are more susceptible to the effects of bile acids than others, and this may be related to the genetics of individual babies. Bile acid levels can also go up and down very quickly, so blood test results may not reflect the bile acid levels a couple of days after the test. In ICP, bile acids cross the placenta and are thought to cause very subtle heart-rate irregularities in the baby.[17] While this is uncommon, it is also unpredictable because ICP babies are otherwise well and show no signs of problems beforehand. Their placentas function well and they often grow larger than average.[14]

There are no consistent guidelines about managing ICP. Medication (ursodeoxycholic acid, UDCA) may help to reduce itching for some women.[18] However, there are currently no antenatal monitoring methods that can adequately assess the wellbeing of the baby, or predict or prevent stillbirth.[18] More recent recommendations focus on monitoring bile acid levels due to the link between levels and complications.[19] Therefore, if women have symptoms, bile acids should be regularly assessed, even if the results are normal.[15] The results of these tests can help to inform decision-making about the timing of birth.

Induction of labour for ICP is recommended due to the increased rate of stillbirth in the final weeks of pregnancy. However, the risks of pre-term birth must be weighed against the risk of stillbirth. Therefore, induction is usually offered between 37 and 38 weeks.[13] The timing of birth should be agreed between the woman and her care provider, taking into consideration bile acid levels and symptoms.

With my first baby I was diagnosed with ICP at 38 weeks with bile acids under 20. I was in for monitoring in the day assessment unit and baby wasn't happy on the CTG monitor. The midwife handled it beautifully and was very calm, she said 'you may be meeting your baby this afternoon', and suggested my husband came in ASAP. She listened to me, and my worries. A lovely obstetrician came and made the final call for me to be admitted for induction. I felt in control. I had a membrane sweep and prostin. The midwife suggested I go walk up and down the stairs sideways as many times as I could, and go for a nice dinner at the hospital café with my husband (our last child-free dinner!), and the contractions started coming! I laboured through the night – my husband had gone home. They wanted to break my waters in the morning, but they were too busy all day. Finally, late afternoon I walked up to the midwives' station, started pushing and said I'd weed my pants and needed to have my baby! I was moved round to the delivery ward and had a beautiful straightforward birth on my back with the bloody CTG monitors.

With my second baby I had not itched during pregnancy but had pain in the upper right side of my abdomen, so I had ICP bloods 'just in case'. My bile acid level was 16. I can never forget how strong the intuition was that my baby needed to be born. I saw a registrar and I said 'What is the plan, and when will I be induced?' He said 'It isn't a serious condition anymore, is there a social reason you want to be induced?' The midwife in the day assessment unit comforted me, and told me everything would be OK, and I could come back the following morning for a second opinion. She made me feel safe, but I was so scared. That night I cried a lot, argued with my husband, found support from the charity ICP Support and read all the research I could find. I arrived back at the hospital at about 9.30am the following morning and I was in some sort of early labour. It took a couple of days until my baby arrived. I needed three doses of prostin, then the midwife did the ARM [artificial rupture of membranes], and I had continuous CTG monitoring. I birthed on all fours on the bed. It was a beautiful birth.   Alice

A growth-restricted baby

The term 'small for gestational age' (SGA) is used to describe a baby whose weight is below the 10th centile for gestational age. For many babies being small is normal and due to genetic factors. However, for some babies SGA is caused by growth restriction called 'intrauterine growth restriction' (IUGR). Growth restriction occurs when the placenta is not functioning effectively, and there is reduced transfer of oxygen and nutrients to the baby. This can be caused by a number of factors including pre-eclampsia, an undernourished mother, substance abuse and severe anaemia. Babies who are growth restricted are at increased risk of stillbirth, infant death and disability. However, the risk reduces significantly for babies diagnosed with IUGR in pregnancy.[20] For example, the rate of stillbirth is 1.9% of births for babies with IUGR that is not identified before birth. The stillbirth rate for babies who are diagnosed with IUGR in pregnancy is 0.9%. Therefore it is important to identify IUGR babies in pregnancy to help improve their outcomes.

The diagnosis of IUGR cannot be made based only on estimating the size and weight of a baby. Ultrasound estimations of babies' weights are not very accurate, and can be more than 10% higher or lower than the actual weight.[21] In addition, ultrasound weight estimation cannot distinguish between normal SGA babies, and IUGR babies. Diagnosing IUGR requires a more detailed assessment of how well the placenta is functioning. This assessment is carried out using an ultrasound Doppler to measure the blood flow through the umbilical cord to the baby.[22] This is different to the Doppler used to listen to the baby's heart rate during an antenatal appointment, and requires an ultrasound machine. An umbilical Doppler is the only evidence-based method of determining the wellbeing of the baby, and provides a good assessment of how the placenta is functioning.[23]

Unfortunately, there is no effective intervention to improve the placental function of an IUGR baby. Therefore, the birth of the baby is usually recommended before the function of the placenta declines further. Decisions about the timing of birth need to take into consideration the risks of pre-term birth compared to the risks of continuing the pregnancy with a poorly functioning placenta. The Royal College of

Obstetricians and Gynaecologists recommends that IUGR babies with abnormal Doppler assessments should be born urgently, even if they are pre-term.[23] However, they also recommend that mothers with SGA babies with normal Doppler assessments should be offered 'delivery' at 37 weeks.

IUGR babies are at an increased risk of distress during labour.[23] This is due to the effect of contractions on a placenta that is not functioning effectively. Every labour contraction interrupts the blood supply through the placenta temporarily. Normally, a healthy placenta can compensate for this in between contractions. However, a placenta that already has a reduced blood supply may be unable to adequately support the baby through labour. In addition, an IUGR baby will often have lower amniotic fluid than a well-grown baby; and amniotic fluid protects the baby from contractions during labour (see page 89). The problems that IUGR babies have in labour can be worse with an induced labour where the contractions tend to be stronger than spontaneous contractions (see chapter 6). There have been no recent studies examining the outcomes for IUGR babies following induced or spontaneous labour. However, old studies reported that during labour 75-95% of IUGR babies required a caesarean due to signs of distress.[23] Therefore, NICE guidelines recommend that induction of labour is not appropriate for babies with severe IUGR.[24] In these cases, a planned caesarean will likely result in better outcomes for the baby.

With my first baby I had an awesome pregnancy. I planned to go into labour naturally, and was aiming for a drug-free, calm birth. The universe had other ideas! The 36-week scan identified that baby's tummy growth had slowed. At 37 weeks it had improved. At 38 weeks it had plateaued again. They wanted to induce on the spot. I said 'No', and asked to go home. I was scared and anxious and angry (and in denial) all at the same time. I went back the following day for a stretch and sweep and started having irregular surges through the weekend. On Monday we arrived at the hospital for a check-up at 8am and it all went downhill from there basically. I refused induction until after 1pm, based on the fact that all monitoring was showing him as happy and healthy. Eventually they wore me down and we agreed. Once syntocinon was commenced my cervix dilated to 8cm in two hours. There were concerns about my baby's heart rate and I ended up having an emergency caesarean under general anaesthetic. Lewis was born weighing 2.4kg [5lbs 3oz]. Apgar scores of 1 and 6, but he recovered really well and is the most beautiful little boy and we are very lucky.   Rachel

When I was informed by the obstetric sonographer that Tom was significantly growth restricted at a third trimester scan I was in shock and the tears welled up very quickly! Having vaginally birthed two healthy girls previously, I had never had complications like this before. I was quickly referred to the hospital and it was recommended I birth my little one in the next couple of days – I was 34 weeks pregnant. The doctors and midwives explored all the options with me, and were very respectful. As he was lying transverse [sideways], and was quite compromised already, I chose to have a caesarean section. For us that was the right choice. Being a midwife myself, I was aware that Tom would have really struggled with an induction due to the limited blood flow through my placenta. This was not at all what I had imagined when I was planning his birth months earlier, however it was absolutely the right decision, and it was a beautiful, calm, gentle birth for him and he was in very good condition at birth. I had skin-to-skin in the operating theatre and even got to choose which music was playing while *he was born. All the health professionals involved recommended different options, but ultimately I knew it was my choice in how Tom was born and I have no regrets with choosing to birth via caesarean.*   *Lauren*

Reduced fetal movements

Women usually start to feel their baby moving between 16 and 20 weeks' gestation. These movements change during pregnancy, increasing in strength as the baby grows. The number of movements a baby makes tends to increase progressively until about 32 weeks.[25] From 32 weeks on, the frequency of movements usually remains consistent until labour starts. There is no evidence to support the idea that movements decrease as pregnancy advances, or prior to the onset of labour.[26] The term 'reduced fetal movements' (RFM) refers to a baby who is making smaller movements, or fewer movements, than is usual for them.

The use of movement counting, or 'kick-charts' to assess babies' wellbeing is not supported by evidence, and this type of monitoring has been found to increase women's anxiety levels.[25] Women become familiar with their own baby's individual movement patterns during pregnancy, and are the best judge as to whether there has been a change in movement. In addition, a mother's intuition should be listened to regarding baby's wellbeing. Significant changes should be reported to care providers and investigated. This can include a reduction in movements, a sudden alteration in the type of movement, or feelings of concern about the baby's wellbeing. Tests to assess the wellbeing of the baby will depend on the gestation, but may include monitoring the baby's heart rate with a CTG (cardiotocograph) machine; an ultrasound assessment of the baby's size and amniotic fluid level; and an ultrasound Doppler assessment of blood flow through the placenta.[25]

RFM is common, with 40% of women reporting RFM at some point during their pregnancy.[26] RFM can be caused by a number of harmless factors, such as the position of the baby, or the position of the placenta. After one episode of RFM there is a 70% chance that there will be no further complications.[26] Therefore, induction is not recommended for a single episode of RFM if the pregnancy remains otherwise healthy.[25] However, women who experience recurrent episodes of RFM during pregnancy are at increased risk of complications, including growth restriction (see above), preterm labour, congenital abnormalities and stillbirth.[26] RFM can be a sign that the baby is not getting adequate oxygen through the placenta, and is therefore slowing movements to conserve energy. There are no studies assessing whether induction reduces the risk of complications for women with recurrent RFM. Therefore, the Royal College of Obstetricians and Gynaecologists recommends that the decision about inducing labour for recurrent RFM should be made taking into account other factors, such as whether the baby is IUGR, and the pros and cons of induction for the individual woman.[25] In addition, if RFM is due to problems with the placenta, the baby may encounter the same problems in labour as an IUGR baby (see above).

I was induced with my third child. I was 36+5 weeks and she had stopped moving. I made the decision along with my midwife, my husband and the medical team at the hospital, following a week of close monitoring and ultrasounds for reduced fetal movements. I knew the importance of fetal movements and, from my experience as a midwife, I have seen the potential tragic consequences of ignoring changes in fetal movements. I felt well informed and confident in my decision to go ahead with induction. My membranes were artificially ruptured at 3pm, a syntocinon drip was started at 5pm, I established labour at 6pm and she was born at 8.25pm. I had a vaginal birth of a healthy baby girl weighing 2.6kg [5lb 7oz] with Apgars of 9. I was terrified of being induced, and was worried that we were making the wrong decision, considering that my daughter would be a little bit premature. But it turned out to be exactly the right decision as, when she was born, she was very tangled up in her short cord, so that was thought to be the cause of the RFM. If we'd left things to carry on until full term, we could've potentially had a much worse outcome.   Samantha L

Prolonged pre-term rupture of membranes

Prolonged pre-term rupture of membranes (P-PROM) refers to the amniotic sac breaking before 37 weeks' gestation without further signs of labour. If the amniotic sac breaks at 37 weeks or later, it is considered a variation of labour rather than a complication (see page 79). Most women with P-PROM will go on to experience pre-term labour in the following 24 hours.[27]

The risks of P-PROM are mostly due to the complications associated with pre-term birth for the baby. Therefore, the closer to 37 weeks the pregnancy is, the better the likely outcome for the baby. However, the amniotic sac protects the baby from infection during pregnancy, and P-PROM can be caused by an infection damaging the amniotic sac membrane. Once the membranes are broken there is a risk of infection of the amniotic fluid and also the baby. Giving women with P-PROM antibiotics reduces the chance of pre-term labour, and reduces the chance of infection-related complications for the baby after birth.[28]

In the past, induction of labour for P-PROM has been recommended to reduce the risk of infection for the baby. However, a recent Cochrane review does not support this approach.[29] The review compared early planned birth (by induction or planned caesarean) for P-PROM with waiting for spontaneous labour, and found no difference in the rates of infection. Early planned birth was associated with increased rates of breathing difficulties for the baby, admission to special care nursery and increased risk of death. The review concluded that for women with P-PROM before 37 weeks, waiting for spontaneous labour, with careful monitoring, improves outcomes for the mother and baby.

I had pre-term rupture of membranes at 36 weeks with my first baby with no prior risk factors. After 10 hours and contractions being 2–3 minutes apart with minimal cervical dilation, a doctor appeared and informed us that they would be 'putting me on a drip to speed things up'. No other reason whatsoever and no discussion. My labour actually slowed at this point. My midwife refused induction on my behalf, and requested they give me more time to labour on my own. After another 11 hours of mostly undisturbed labour, I delivered my baby un-medicated and without intervention. I'm really thankful that my midwife advocated for me at the time. I was quite taken back by how abrupt the doctor was, and that I had no apparent choice in the matter even though I did not want to be induced. As a first time mum it was extremely confusing, and a bit intimidating just being 'told' by someone I didn't know. Without my midwife, I know my birth would have been a very different and not a necessarily pleasant experience. Rebecca

The death of a baby

When a baby dies before birth, it can be extremely difficult to make decisions about how to birth the baby while grappling with shock, devastation and grief. There is usually no need to rush decisions about birth, and the woman may wish to go home and spend some time with her family before making a decision about when, or how to birth her baby. Support groups such as SANDS (Stillbirth and Neonatal Death Charity) can also offer support during this time (see page 154).

In most cases a vaginal birth is preferable to a caesarean due to the risks of surgery for the woman. If there is no bleeding or infection, and if the amniotic sac is still intact, there is no reason why the woman cannot wait for spontaneous labour.[24] However, many women choose to be induced when their baby dies. Planning when the birth will happen can help women to organise the support they need around them during and after labour. The induction process for a stillborn baby differs because there are no concerns about the effect of medications on the baby. For example, induction methods may include an oral medication to induce contractions in addition to the usual methods. Very strong pain relief medication can also be given to women during labour.

A woman who has experienced a stillbirth is at an increased risk of having a stillbirth in a subsequent pregnancy (2.5% compared to 0.4% for women with no history of stillbirth).[30] Therefore, induction is often offered to women who have experienced the loss of a baby in a previous pregnancy.

On May 20, 2005, at 40 weeks and 5 days gestation, we found out that our second daughter had unexpectedly died in utero, and would subsequently be stillborn. My obstetrician recommended induction as I had had a previous uncomplicated spontaneous vaginal birth. My husband, however, was keen for me to have a caesarean section, as he couldn't stand the thought of seeing me go through the physical pain of labour and birth, as well as the emotional pain of stillbirth. A caesarean section did not even cross my mind; nor did waiting to go into spontaneous labour. At that stage I felt that I had held on to my baby for long enough in utero, and I needed to now hold her in my arms, and also share her with others for the short time that we had to say our hellos and goodbyes. Later that evening I was given prostin and some sleeping tablets. After a fitful night's sleep, the next morning I had an ARM [artificial rupture of membranes] *and elected to have an early epidural sited prior to the commencement of the syntocinon drip. I didn't really know what to expect with either the induction, or birthing a stillborn baby. Both scenarios were so frighteningly foreign to me. My vague memories of the labour are that it was surprisingly calm and relatively painless. I used the PCEA* [patient controlled epidural anaesthesia] *with good effect, and after a five-hour labour I had quite a quick birth. The birth was also surprisingly calm and peaceful, though so very quiet at the end when my dear, limp, pale, and bloody beautiful 8lb 3oz* [3.7kg] *baby Annabelle was placed in my arms. If I had my time over again, there is no question that I would give anything to have Annabelle alive, breathing and kicking; however, over time I have accepted that her life was only meant to be the 40 weeks she spent warm, loved and nourished within my womb. I would not change anything about her labour and birth, apart from being able to re-live it over and over and over...*

My next two pregnancies ended with D&Cs [dilation and curettage] *for missed miscarriages. Then I had another induction at 17 weeks for another IUFD* [intrauterine fetal death]. *Elijah was my sixth pregnancy. Understandably, this pregnancy was fraught with anxiety, however this baby (we didn't know the sex) was a very active baby, so I constantly felt reassured that all was going to be OK. Having said that, I was keen to have the baby out sooner rather than later, and so an induction was scheduled for 37 weeks. I know some people (who were more anxious than I was at the time!) were questioning my lack of desire to press my obstetrician for an induction even sooner than 37 weeks. However, when this baby was born, I needed to have him/her in my arms, and with me at all times, not in an isolette in a special care nursery. Even though I had previously experienced an induction, it did feel rather odd presenting to have a baby without being in active labour. It felt strangely similar to checking in to a hotel! As with my previous induction, I was given prostin that evening and had an ARM early the next morning. No time for an epidural this time! ARM at 6.45am, syntocinon infusion commenced at 7.30am, syntocinon turned down at 7.50am, syntocinon off at 8.00am, and baby born at 8.50am! In retrospect, there was probably no need for the syntocinon. Although at the time the labour felt fast and intense, it was also over too quickly to remember too much. Not having an epidural this time, I felt absolutely fabulous after the birth, being able to get up and shower, and walk around almost immediately (after a beautiful delicious first breastfeed of course). And the joy of FINALLY having another newborn baby in my arms: there are no words to describe this feeling.*   *Paula*

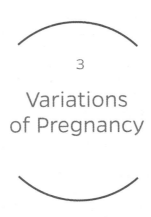

3

Variations
of Pregnancy

Many inductions of labour are carried out due to variations in pregnancy. In these cases the mother and baby are both well, but the pregnancy variation increases the chance of particular complications occurring. Making a decision about induction for a variation involves comparing the possible but unlikely complications associated with that variation, with the risks of induction. This chapter discusses the main variations of pregnancy that result in women being offered induction. Research, guidelines, and women's experiences are discussed to help readers to make their own decisions about induction in their individual situation. A lot of the research focuses on how variations alter the general 'perinatal death' rate. The term 'perinatal death' refers to the death of a baby before, or soon after birth. The range of time covered by this term is usually from 22 weeks' gestation until seven days after birth. Therefore, the perinatal death rate includes stillbirth and early infant death. Perinatal death is uncommon in well-resourced countries: for example, in the United Kingdom, the general perinatal death rate from all causes is 0.65%.[1]

Post-dates and post-term pregnancy

A pregnancy is considered to be 'term' between 37 and 42 weeks after the first day of the last menstrual period. Once a pregnancy progresses beyond 42 weeks, it is referred to as 'post-term'. However, few pregnancies reach 42 weeks because induction of labour is usually carried out when a pregnancy is 'post-dates' to prevent it from becoming 'post-term'. A post-dates pregnancy is simply one that has continued beyond the estimated due date (EDD). The recommended timing for induction differs between maternity services, but is usually after 41 weeks.

Before modern science, women used the moon's cycle to track their menstrual cycles and to estimate when their babies would be born.[2] Women expected to give birth within 10 moon cycles after their last monthly bleed. The moon cycle is 29.5 days, and 10 moon cycles takes 295 days, or 42 weeks to complete. Since the 1700s attempts have been made to estimate specific due dates for all babies. This idea was underpinned by the development of science, and an understanding of the body as a machine with definable, measurable parts and processes, of which pregnancy was one.[3] The formula created in the 1700s to estimate a due date is still used today, and is based on the assumption that birth takes place 40 weeks (280 days) after the first day of the last monthly period (LMP).[4] In the last decade, 'dating' ultrasound scans have been routinely offered to women at 10–13 weeks' gestation. Dating scans attempt to calculate the gestational age of the baby and, based on that, estimate the date on which the baby will be 40 weeks. However, EDDs based on ultrasounds (at any gestation) are no more accurate than EDDs based on a reliable LMP date,[5] and neither method provides an accurate due date.

Research has clearly shown that the average pregnancy does not last 40 weeks, and only 35% of women give birth during the week of their EDD.[5] For women having their first baby, pregnancy lasts on average 40 weeks and 5 days; and 75% will give birth spontaneously by 41 weeks and 2 days.[6] For women having their second (or more) baby, the average pregnancy lasts 40 weeks and 3 days; and 75% will give birth spontaneously by 41 weeks.

A number of other factors are known to influence how long an individual woman's pregnancy will last. Women's bodies are unique, and there is wide variation in how a pregnancy develops from conception to birth. For example, ovulation does not always occur on day 14, even in menstrual cycles that are 28 days long.[7] An embryo that takes longer to implant into the uterus, will take longer to gestate.[8] Even a woman's diet may influence the length of her pregnancy.[9] However, the most important factor appears to be genetics,[4] and longer pregnancies literally run in families. A baby will take longer to gestate if their mother, or their father, comes from a family with longer pregnancies. A woman who has her first baby after the EDD is very likely to have her subsequent babies after the EDD.[10]

Induction for post-dates

Induction for a post-dates pregnancy is primarily offered because the general rate of perinatal death (stillbirth and early infant death) increases after 42 weeks. While the increase is statistically significant, the rate remains under 1%. For example, the perinatal death rate is around 0.1% at 40–41 weeks, 0.3% at 42 weeks and 0.5% after 43 weeks.[11] A Cochrane review found that induction of labour before 42 weeks reduced the perinatal death rate from 0.3% to 0.03%.[12] This finding is the primary reason for recommending induction for all women with post-dates pregnancies.

The reason for the slight increase in the perinatal death rate in post-dates pregnancies is unknown. Current research focuses on general outcomes, on 'what' happens rather than 'why' or 'how'. In the absence of a clear answer, many care providers believe that the placenta deteriorates after 41 weeks, and is therefore less able to provide adequate nutrients and oxygen to the baby. There is evidence that the structure and biochemistry of the placenta changes as pregnancy develops. Some scientists interpret these changes as the placenta growing and adapting to meet the changing needs of the baby.[13] Others suggest that these changes are due to the aging and deterioration of the placenta.[14] However, tests of placental function show no changes in post-dates pregnancies.[15] In addition, most babies continue to grow after 40 weeks, suggesting that they continue to receive adequate nutrients and oxygen. The studies that identify an increased perinatal death rate for post-dates pregnancies do not identify the placenta as a problem.[12] Another possibility is that the increased death rate may be due to problems with the baby, or the pregnancy that cause a delay in spontaneous labour, rather than the other way around. The Cochrane review found that a third of the perinatal deaths reported in the studies reviewed were due to pre-existing congenital abnormalities.

For the vast majority of women, a post-dates pregnancy is a normal and healthy individual variation. However, it is difficult for individual women to determine if their post-dates pregnancy is normal for them, or whether they will experience a rare complication. If a woman has previously experienced a post-dates pregnancy without complications, there is no increased risk of perinatal death, or any other type of complication if they wait for spontaneous labour.[10] If the woman has not previously had a post-dates pregnancy, it might help to consider what is a normal gestation within her family.

Baby number four was born at 41+5. I chose induction (in hindsight) as I had some internal emotional factors that were holding me back from letting things progress. After trying all the natural methods of induction, I decided it was time to get things really going. A few times I had pressure from the obstetrician to induce, but I had a supportive midwife happy to go along with my decision. I had minimal fetal movement by 41 weeks, so daily monitoring was required, but all was okay. By 41+2 weeks I had my first stretch and sweep. I begged the obstetrician to do an ARM [artificial rupture of membranes], but to no avail. 41+5 weeks rolled around, and I finally went in for induction! My waters were broken, and I walked the stairs, and got things really going within two hours. Five hours after the ARM, I sent everyone out of the room as I felt I wasn't in the zone and 'I had to get my shit together'. I had a vaginal examination as I was feeling pushy, and things didn't seem to be progressing as quick as I had hoped for (I was 6cm dilated at the time). My baby was born 20 minutes later, with only my midwife and a student in the room. Samantha D

At 40+10 we had a scan. Fluid levels were great and baby was measuring fine. I was informed that induction was the safest option despite there being no risks other than we were past my due date. At 40+12 my membranes were ruptured in the hospital, and my body went into early labour. I asked for time to see what my body would do, but after two hours I was told the syntocinon was necessary. I had contractions, one on top of the other, for a couple of hours, then pushed for a couple more before being told I was too exhausted, and that I had half an hour to keep trying before the obstetrician was coming to deliver my baby. My baby was delivered half an hour later by the obstetrician with forceps. She was still covered in vernix with Apgars of 9 and 9. My thoughts about it now – having had my second baby as a spontaneous natural delivery, and understanding what labour can be like – I feel robbed for what I experienced with my firstborn and still feel a lot of sadness when I think about it. *Meg*

Spontaneous post-dates labour

Around 90% of women who choose to wait for spontaneous labour will give birth before 42 weeks, and only 1% will remain pregnant beyond 43 weeks.[12] Most guidelines recommend additional monitoring of the baby's wellbeing from 42 weeks. This involves monitoring the baby's heart rate with a CTG (cardiotocograph) machine, and measuring the amniotic fluid with ultrasound. However, no form of antenatal monitoring reduces the chance of complications.[12] Women also need to consider the impact of antenatal monitoring on their experience of waiting. Some women find that monitoring raises anxiety, especially when low amniotic fluid volume is identified. Amniotic fluid often reduces after 40 weeks, so this is a common finding in post-dates pregnancies. Anxiety and stress can interfere with oxytocin release and potentially delay the onset of labour (see chapter 4). In contrast, other women find monitoring reassuring, despite the fact that monitoring does not improve outcomes. For these women, monitoring can reduce stress and assist with oxytocin release. The best indicator of a baby's wellbeing is their movement (see page 51). Women with concerns about their baby's wellbeing should be encouraged to pay close attention to their baby's movements, regardless of whether they choose additional monitoring or not.

There are a few factors associated with post-dates pregnancies that may alter the experience of spontaneous labour. Post-dates babies tend to be bigger because they continue to grow in the final weeks of pregnancy (see 'suspected big baby' below). However, big babies rarely cause problems during labour unless the woman also has poorly managed gestational diabetes (see page 36). As mentioned above, there may be lower levels of amniotic fluid after 40 weeks. During labour, amniotic fluid protects the baby, placenta and umbilical cord from compression during contractions (see chapter 4). However, a healthy post-dates baby can cope well with some compression during contractions, particularly if there is enough time between contractions to recover. Spontaneous labour contractions tend to be more spaced out, and gentler in comparison to induced contractions (see chapter 6). In an induced labour there is even less amniotic fluid because the induction process involves breaking the amniotic sac to release the fluid (see chapter 5). The lack of amniotic fluid, along with stronger induced contractions, increases the chance that the baby will become distressed.

The amniotic sac usually breaks towards the end of a spontaneous labour (see chapter 4), and in a post-dates labour there is likely to be meconium in the fluid. Meconium is made up of mostly water, and a number of substances including amniotic fluid and intestinal cells. At the end of pregnancy the baby's bowels are full of meconium, which is passed in the baby's stools during the first days after birth. Meconium-stained amniotic fluid is normal and common in a post-dates labour because the baby's digestive system is mature and begins to function before birth, passing meconium into the amniotic fluid. Meconium-stained amniotic fluid occurs in 30–40% of pregnancies after 42 weeks.[16] There is a theory that meconium-stained fluid indicates a baby is severely distressed. However, the connection between meconium and distress has not been proven. Most babies who become distressed in labour do not pass meconium, and most babies who pass meconium in labour show no signs of distress.[16] Nevertheless, based on this theory, all babies that are known to have passed meconium are treated as if they are potentially distressed.

Many care providers believe that meconium-stained fluid can cause a condition called 'meconium aspiration syndrome' (MAS). MAS is thought to occur when a baby inhales meconium-stained amniotic fluid into their lungs during labour, resulting in problems with breathing and/or infection after birth. However, a baby will only inhale deeply enough to get fluid into their lungs if the oxygen supply through their placenta drops to extremely low levels for a long period of time. This situation is unlikely to go undetected if the baby's heart-rate is being listened to regularly during labour. The diagnosis of MAS is controversial, because the symptoms of MAS can also be found in babies who did not have meconium-stained fluid.[17] This leads some researchers to question whether the symptoms are caused by meconium, or whether meconium happens to be present at the same time as symptoms.[17] MAS is more likely to be diagnosed in babies born after 41 weeks (0.7%), compared to babies induced before 41 weeks.[12] However, there is no difference in the rate of admission to special care nursery between babies born after a spontaneous labour compared to an induced labour. This suggests that post-dates babies who have problems at birth are diagnosed with MAS because meconium is present, whereas induced babies with the same problems are given a different diagnosis.

Many hospital guidelines recommend the use of a CTG machine to continuously monitor the baby's heart rate during post-dates labours. Guidelines also recommend continuous monitoring if meconium fluid is seen, regardless of gestation. These recommendations are based on common practice, rather than on research evidence. CTG machines are not very accurate at assessing whether a baby is distressed or not. In most cases where the CTG trace is classified as 'abnormal', the baby is fine.[18] Therefore, CTG monitoring increases a woman's chance of having a caesarean significantly, without improving the outcome for her baby.[19] National Institute for Health and Care Excellence (NICE) guidelines recommend that care providers should not offer CTG monitoring to women with 'non-significant' meconium-stained liquor unless there are other risk factors.[20] Non-significant refers to the normal yellow-coloured light meconium staining. Significant meconium includes the presence of dark green or black, thick or lumpy meconium. Instead, NICE recommend that care providers should listen to the baby's heart-rate regularly using a hand-held device, and only put the CTG on if any problems are identified.

At 42 weeks with my first baby, my midwife advised that an induction should be considered. I was planning a home birth, felt well, baby was moving well, and I saw no need to change plans and risk a cascade of interventions. I knew my body wasn't ready yet, so the only option I was happy with was to wait. Sure, I wanted to meet my baby, but I didn't want the risks associated with induction. I went into labour at 43 weeks and had a lengthy pre-labour. My waters broke as I got into established labour and I didn't recognise the pale yellow as meconium until later. By the time my midwife came over I was in the pool and the lighting was dim. Baby's heart rate was great so we weren't concerned. My daughter was born at home at 43+1 weeks, and she had no problems after she was born.

I felt strong and powerful, on top of the world, like I could do anything. *Anna*

I was induced with my first child in hospital at 10 days past 40 weeks for 'post dates' (scoff). I felt like I had no rights over my body and baby, and it was a horribly traumatic experience for me. I suffered postnatal depression and post-traumatic stress disorder afterwards. I then went on to have three incredible home births at 43+1, 42+5 and 44 weeks. I had meconium in my waters when they broke with my third pregnancy. Funnily enough, after this happened my labour completely stopped, directly in response to my fear. That was until my midwife got to my house, and listened to the baby's heartbeat, which was strong – then labour began again, in full force and she was born 70 minutes later. When she was born there was no meconium on her and she wriggled her entire way out of me – kicking even as she was crowning. I think looking back it was my baby's way of telling me and reassuring me that all was well. *Jessica*

Advanced maternal age

In maternity care the term 'advanced maternal age' is used to refer to a pregnant woman who is 35 or over. In 2016, 22% of women giving birth in the United Kingdom were over 35.[21] The general rate of stillbirth increases for women over 35 once their pregnancy progresses beyond 39 weeks. For example, women over 40 years old have a 0.2% chance of stillbirth at 39–40 weeks, compared to a 0.1% chance for women under 35 years old. While this rise is statistically significant, the rate of stillbirth remains low regardless of age or gestation. For example, a woman over 40 years old, and 42 weeks pregnant, has a 1% chance of stillbirth.[22] The reason for the increased rate of stillbirth is not known. Older mothers, in general, are more likely to have complicated pregnancies, and/or babies with congenital abnormalities.[23] However, even when these factors are taken into consideration, the stillbirth rate remains higher for women over 35 compared to younger women.[23] There is also no evidence that routine assessments of babies' growth or wellbeing will improve outcomes.[23]

Based on the general risk of stillbirth, The Royal College of Obstetricians and Gynaecologists (RCOG) recommends induction at 39 weeks for women who are 40 years old or older.[23] Since the recommendation was published, a study has looked at the outcomes of induction of labour for women 35 and older.[24] The study found no significant difference in the perinatal death rate for women induced at 39 weeks, compared to women who remained pregnant. However, in this study induction of labour at 40 weeks reduced the perinatal death rate from 0.26% to 0.08%. The researchers concluded that perinatal death is rare, even for women aged 35 and over, and that 562 inductions would need to be carried out at 40 weeks to prevent one death. The study also found that induction before 41 weeks was associated with a 20–30% increased rate of emergency caesarean, and a 10% increased rate of instrumental delivery (vacuum or forceps). Women and babies were also more likely to be re-admitted to hospital within 28 days of the birth after induction of labour.

At my first antenatal appointment with my back-up hospital (I was planning a freebirth), I was informed that, because I would be 41 years of age by the time my baby would be born, I would be booked in for an induction at 40 weeks. I asked the student doctor to present me with the relevant studies and evidence as to why this policy was in place. He couldn't. I declined because I believed the policy was a broad spectrum, one size fits all, intervention. My baby was born at 43 weeks.   *Lynda*

Vaginal birth after caesarean

In the United Kingdom around 26% of women give birth by caesarean.[25] Many of these women go on to have another pregnancy, and need to decide whether to plan another caesearean, or plan a vaginal birth after caesarean (VBAC). The primary risk associated with VBAC is uterine rupture, which occurs when the previous caesearean scar tears. This is a rare complication, occurring in less than 0.5% of VBAC labours.[26] This rate may be higher for women who have had more than one caesearean, at around 0.9%.[27] In most cases of uterine rupture, the complication is identified and managed by an emergency caesearean, and 94% of babies survive this experience. The chance of stillbirth and infant death during a VBAC labour is extremely low, and comparable to the risk of a woman having her first baby with no caesarean scar. Women who plan a VBAC have a 75% chance of having a vaginal birth, which is higher than a woman having her first baby.[26]

The alternative to a VBAC, a repeat planned caesarean, also carries risks.[28] For example, there are a number of complications that can occur with a caesearean, including bleeding resulting in hysterectomy (0.7%); bladder or bowel injury (0.1%); infection (6%); readmission to hospital (5%) and persistent pain in the first few months (9%). Around 1–2% of babies born by caesarean are accidentally cut during the procedure. Labour prepares the baby for the transition to life outside the uterus (see chapter 4). Babies who do not experience labour are more likely to have breathing problems at birth requiring admission to special care.[29] They also miss out on being exposed to vaginal bacteria, resulting in a different gut microbiome.[30] This may explain why babies born by caesarean section are more likely to have health problems, such as asthma and diabetes, later in life.[31] A repeat caesarean also increases the chance of complications in future pregnancies, such as an abnormally attached placenta

(0.6%) and an increased stillbirth rate (0.4% compared with 0.2% following a vaginal birth).[26]

Women planning a VBAC can experience pressure from their care providers to go into labour before 40 weeks. This is based on an increased rate of stillbirth (0.11%) from 39 weeks onwards in comparison to women who have not had a previous caesarean (0.05%).[26] However, most women do not go into spontaneous labour until after 40 weeks (see 'post-dates and post-term pregnancy' above). Many women had their caesarean during an induction for a post-dates pregnancy, which suggests that a longer gestation is normal for them. The start of spontaneous labour may also be inhibited by stress and anxiety about giving birth within a particular timeframe (see chapter 4).

Despite the preferences of individual care providers, RCOG and NICE do not support earlier induction for women planning a VBAC.[26, 32] Instead, they recommend that induction be offered at 41 weeks, the same gestation as for non-VBAC women. However, there are additional risks associated with induction of labour after a previous caesarean. The chance of a uterine rupture increases from 0.5% to 1%, and the chance of an emergency caesarean increases to 37% compared to 26% during a spontaneous VBAC labour.[26] There is evidence that this is mostly caused by syntocinon used during induction and, less commonly, prostin (see chapter 4 and 6). Therefore, RCOG and NICE do not recommend the use of syntocinon during a VBAC labour, and recommend using only low doses of prostin.[26, 36] Alternatively, mechanical methods of induction, such as balloon catheters, can be used (see chapter 5), or women can wait for spontaneous labour.

As baby number one ended up as an emergency caesarean, baby number two was a VBAC attempt. I did all my research

on everything. My hospital didn't offer induction for VBACs –
it was go into labour naturally, or automatic caesarean. They
tried from the very start to book in my caesarean date for 10 days
over. I declined at every appointment. My MGP [midwifery
group practice] *midwife told me that I could still opt for an*
induction if I wanted – she had seen successful VBACs with
induction (balloon catheter etc.) – regardless of policy. All my
research led me to decide to simply wait. No caesarean booked
in for 39 weeks, no automatic caesarean at 40+10 for being late.
Baby was born 12 days 'late' – via VBAC with no intervention,
and to the horror of all the obstetricians who bullied me at every
turn to do what suited them.   *Kimberley*

A VBAC induction was discussed with me. I simply stated
that I would have further monitoring at 42 weeks, and make
a plan from there. I was booked into a couple of hospitals;
one was fine with this approach. The other assumed that I'd
simply book a repeat caesarean if I got to this point. I ended up
birthing at home at 41 weeks.   *Helen*

Suspected big baby

A baby weighing 8lb 13oz (4kg) or more is considered to be
'big' (macrosomic). In the United Kingdom more than 10%
of babies weigh over 8lb 13oz at birth.[33] The term 'large for
gestational age' is used to describe a baby who is on the 90th
percentile at birth, meaning that the baby is bigger than 90%
of other babies born at that gestation. The only way of determining
the weight of a baby is to weigh them after birth. There is no
accurate method of estimating the size of a baby before birth.
Estimating the size of a baby by palpating and measuring a
woman's pregnant bump is incorrect more than 50% of the
time,[34] because factors such as the woman's individual anatomy,
and the baby's position, alter measurements.

The best available method of assessing a baby's weight before birth involves measuring the baby's abdomen with ultrasound.[35] However, this method only predicts the weight of the baby within 15% of their actual weight. For example, if a baby's actual weight was 8lb, the ultrasound estimation could be anywhere between 6lbs 13oz and 9lb 3oz. The inaccuracy of weight estimation results in many women being incorrectly told they are pregnant with a big baby. A study in the United States found that two out of three pregnant women were told their baby was 'too big' according to ultrasound.[36] In this study the average birth weight of the babies estimated to be 'big' was 7lb 13oz.

The size of a baby is influenced by a number of factors, including genetics. Big babies tend to run in families, and many women will naturally grow a big, healthy baby. In addition, babies continue to grow throughout pregnancy, so a baby born at 42 weeks will be bigger than he or she would have been at 40 weeks. Therefore, having a big baby can be healthy and normal for an individual woman. However, abnormal blood glucose levels can also cause a baby to grow bigger, for example if the woman has uncontrolled gestational diabetes. Babies who have grown big due to high blood glucose are a different shape to genetically big babies. Their shoulders and chest are larger and fatter, and they are more likely to encounter complications at birth due to their size and shape. Unfortunately, research into big babies often combines the outcomes for diabetic and non-diabetic women. Therefore, it can be difficult to assess risks for a big baby who is the result of a healthy pregnancy.

Babies who are in the 91st to 97th percentiles have a lower risk of stillbirth (0.1%) in comparison to smaller babies (% varies according to gestation).[37] However, very large babies in the 98th centile have an increased chance of stillbirth (2%).

This may be because babies in the 98th centile are more likely to have a diabetic mother and/or have congenital abnormalities. Birthing a big baby is associated with complications such as severe perineal tearing (0.6%) and postpartum haemorrhage (1.7%).[38] Big babies are also more likely to have low blood glucose at birth (1.2%); temporary rapid breathing (1.5%); and a high temperature (0.6%).[39] However, the main concern care providers have about big babies is the risk of shoulder dystocia. Shoulder dystocia occurs when the baby's shoulders become stuck in the pelvis after the head is born, resulting in a delay in the birth of the body. Care providers may need to assist the woman into positions to release the baby's shoulders, and in some cases they may need to move the baby's shoulders with their fingers. This can be a traumatic experience for mother and baby, and in some cases results in birth injuries. The incidence of shoulder dystocia increases with the size of the baby. For example, it occurs with around 1% of babies weighing less than 8lbs 8oz, compared to 5–9% of babies weighing between 8lb 8oz and 9lb 9oz.[40]

However, the complications associated with big babies may be due to the interventions carried out when a baby is suspected to be big. For example, one study compared the outcomes of a group of women who were suspected to have a big baby, with a group of women who unexpectedly gave birth to a big baby.[41] Women who were suspected of having a big baby were three times more likely to have an induction or caesarean, and were four times more likely to have complications such as severe perineal tearing and postpartum haemorrhage. In this study there were no differences in the incidence of shoulder dystocia between the two groups. Another study found that care providers were more likely to diagnose slow progress during labour and recommend a caesarean if they suspected the baby was big.[42] Women who are told that they have a big baby, and are counselled about potential complications, are significantly more likely to choose a planned caesarean.[43] Therefore, when a baby is suspected of being big, a woman has an increased chance of interventions during birth, and of experiencing complications caused by those interventions, even if the baby is not actually big. The perception of a baby's size influences outcomes more than the actual size of a baby.

Some care providers offer an early induction for a suspected big baby to reduce the chance of shoulder dystocia. A Cochrane review, comparing induction of labour before 40 weeks for a suspected big baby with waiting for spontaneous labour, found that induction decreased the incidence of shoulder dystocia from 6.8% to 4.1%.[44] However, they also found an increased rate of perineal tearing in the induction group of 2.6% compared to 0.7% in the spontaneous labour group, and an increase in the treatment of jaundice for the baby (11% compared to 7%). Therefore, NICE guidelines and World Health Organisation guidelines both state that induction of labour should not be carried out simply because the baby is suspected of being big.[32, 45]

Women can, and do, give birth to big babies without any problems. The physiology of birth involves the mother and baby working together to move the baby through the pelvis safely (see chapter 4). The baby's skull moulds to fit the shape of the mother's pelvis during the slow descent through the vagina. The woman's pelvis can increase in size considerably if she is mobile, and avoids restricting the back of her pelvis by sitting or lying on it. The woman's perineum is capable of stretching without tearing if she follows her instinctive urges to push, and changes position in response to her body. Once the baby's head is born there is a pause as he or she wriggles and rotates their shoulders to move through the pelvis, ready to be born with the next contraction. Interventions that interfere with physiology and instinctive birth, such as an epidural, a reclining birth position, directed pushing and pulling on the baby's head can increase the risk of complications for any baby, especially a big baby.

My obstetrician recommended an induction for my first baby (scheduled for 39 weeks) for suspected macrosomia [big baby]. She told me that a smaller baby would be easier to deliver, and therefore induction was the best thing I could do to avoid a caesarean. For much of the second half of my pregnancy, fundal height measurements had me consistently 2cm or so bigger than 'normal' for gestational age. Palpation suggested my baby was large. I was never given a size scan. Because we have a family history of big babies (my brother was eleven and a quarter pounds!), and all of these babies were birthed vaginally, I was never concerned about a big baby myself. Once my obstetrician became worried about macrosomia, I realised 'her concern' was going to be the bigger problem. But by then, I thought it was too late to seek alternative care for that pregnancy – I proceeded with the induction, trusting my obstetrician's advice, and hoping she was helping me to avoid a caesarean. After 12 hours on syntocinon and dilating to 2–3cm, my induction was deemed a 'failure', and my son was born by caesarean with Apgars of 9 and 10. He was 9lb 4oz [4.2kg].

My obstetrician recommended that all future babies be born by elective rather than unplanned caesarean to avoid 'unpleasantness'. I have since had two more VBAC [vaginal birth after caesarean] babies at home – one at 41+3 weeks who was smaller than my first, and the second at 42+4 weeks. My last baby was bigger than my first and came out with two minutes of pushing, no tears. Tessa

My obstetrician recommended induction with a 'big baby' diagnosis at 37 weeks. I was induced at 39 weeks. No other information was given except 'if we don't induce, baby may get too big and you'll need a caesarean'. I wanted to birth vaginally, but had no idea that diagnosis might be wrong so I accepted it. I had two doses of prostaglandins, and a syntocinon drip. Eventually I had an epidural. They told me to push; I couldn't feel anything, so did nothing. They applied a vacuum on my daughter and kept pulling without contractions. They cut an episiotomy and kept pulling. My baby was born with injuries on her scalp. After all that she was only 3.18kg [7lbs] and 48cm, not big at all. I felt really deceived.   Mariana

Multiple pregnancy

A multiple pregnancy refers to more than one baby growing in the uterus at the same time. Multiple pregnancies are usually twins (two babies), but can be triplets (three babies), quadruplets (four babies) or more. There are also different types of multiple pregnancies. Non-identical (dizygotic) babies are the most common type of multiple pregnancy and result from separate eggs, fertilised by separate sperm. Non-identical babies have a different genetic make-up, and can be different sexes. They also have their own placentas, and are enclosed in their own sac of membranes in the uterus. Identical babies (monozygotic) happen when a single fertilised egg splits, creating more than one baby. Identical babies share the same genetic make-up, and will be the same sex. Depending on when the fertilised egg splits, some identical babies share a placenta and the outside layer of the sac of membranes (the chorion). However, they are usually enclosed in their own inner layer of the membrane sac (the amnion), and therefore remain separated from each other by this thin layer of membrane.

Women who are pregnant with more than one baby have an increased chance of developing complications of pregnancy such as pre-eclampsia and gestational diabetes (see chapter 2). Babies who are multiples are also more likely to be growth restricted and/or be born prematurely. Around 60% of women with twins, and 75% of women with triplets, go into spontaneous labour before 37 weeks.[46] Most of the research into multiple pregnancies focuses on twins rather than triplets or more, because twins are more common. The risk of perinatal death (combined stillbirth and neonatal death) in twin pregnancies increases with gestational age after 37 weeks. For example, the risk of perinatal death at 37 weeks is 0.4% compared to 0.5% at 38 weeks.[47] These general statistics have been used as evidence by NICE guidelines to recommend planned birth, by induction or caesarean, for multiple pregnancies.[46]

The suggested timing of planned birth depends on the type of multiple pregnancy. Birth is recommended from 37 weeks onwards for twins who have their own individual sac of membranes (dichorionic), and from 36 weeks onwards if they share both the inner and outer layer of the membrane sac (monochorionic). For triplets, birth is recommended from 35 weeks. The decision about the type of birth – induction or caesarean – will depend on the position of the babies, and other individual factors.

Despite NICE recommendations, there is little research examining the outcomes of planned early birth for multiple pregnancies. A Cochrane review examined two studies that compared planned birth at 37 weeks for twin pregnancies with waiting for spontaneous labour.[48] There was no difference in the rates of complications, including perinatal death, between the two groups. The WHO guidelines state that there is insufficient evidence to make any recommendation about induction for uncomplicated twin pregnancies.[45]

My third pregnancy was surprise triplets! However, after two previous home births I was determined to give birth vaginally, in hospital, and was forever thankful to my obstetrician who was more than happy for this to happen. As I hit 30 weeks without any previous problems I got sick and started scratching madly. I was diagnosed with cholestasis. I soldiered on through sleepless nights and 3am showers until 32 weeks when I developed gestational diabetes. At 33 weeks I asked my obstetrician for one more week; he obliged. With an induction planned for 8am at 34+6 hanging over my head I decided to get things moving myself to stay away from the cascade of intervention an induction traditionally brings. So the morning of 34+5 I made my husband make love to me, making sure I climaxed too. For the rest of the morning I kept myself busy and did quite a bit of walking. At 1pm my midwife gave me a gentle stretch and sweep; I was 1–2cm dilated at this stage. I sat down just before 8pm with my double electric breast pump. I had planned for 5 minutes pumping; 10 minutes off. The second set of 5 minutes brought on a contraction, and during the third set Baby A's waters broke! I was elated! I pumped once more but contractions were well and truly underway by that stage. I went to hospital within an hour and met my birth team in my labour room. Within 15 minutes Baby A was born, followed by Baby B 11 minutes later and Baby C 3 minutes later! The birth was amazing. I felt in control of my birth for almost the whole time, and it still gives me goosebumps now. To be able to bring them into the world the way I wanted, assisting my body to get into labour was life changing.   *Chenoa*

Pre-labour rupture of membranes after 37 weeks

The amniotic sac plays an important role in the physiology of labour (see chapter 4). Without intervention, the amniotic membranes usually stay intact until close to the end of labour.

However, 10% of women will experience their waters breaking as the first sign of labour, before contractions start. Most of these women (79%) will go into labour within 12 hours of their waters breaking, and 95% will be in spontaneous labour within 24 hours.[49] NICE guidelines recommend offering induction to women who are still not in labour 24 hours after their waters have broken. Induction for pre-labour rupture of membranes is often referred to as 'augmentation' of labour.[32]

The main reason induction is offered after pre-labour rupture of membranes is to reduce the chance of infection for mother and baby. A Cochrane review compared induction for pre-labour rupture of membranes, with waiting for spontaneous labour.[49] Although the review concluded that the rate of infection may be reduced for babies who are induced, it also raised concerns about the low quality of the research. The only finding backed by 'moderate' quality research was that there was no difference in the rate of infant deaths between the induction and waiting groups. The review reported a slight increase (less than 2%) in 'definite and possible' infections for babies when women waited for spontaneous labour. However, once the 'possible' infection results were removed, the difference was no longer significant. The 'possible' infection rate was based on the care provider's observations of symptoms, rather than on clinical diagnosis of infection. For example, if the mother had a raised temperature in labour, her baby may have been assumed to have a possible infection. However, other factors, such as dehydration and epidural analgesia, also increase the temperature of mother and baby during labour. There was also no difference in the Apgar scores of babies in the 'waiting' group, suggesting that babies were well when they were born. Infected babies are more likely to have low Apgar scores and require resuscitation at birth. Babies were more likely to be admitted to special care after a spontaneous labour, but their outcomes were not different in comparison to the induced group of babies. This finding most likely reflects hospital policies that often require routine admission to special care for 'observation' after prolonged rupture of membranes. The review also found a slight increase (1%) in the chance of an infection in the uterus for mothers who waited for labour. The conclusion of the review warns that in order to make a good comparison of outcomes '... evidence about longer-term effects [of induction or waiting] on children is needed.'

Some care providers recommend routine antibiotics for women who have pre-labour rupture of membranes, especially if the baby is not born within a particular timeframe. However, a Cochrane review concluded that antibiotics should not be given routinely to women with ruptured membranes unless there are signs of infection.[50] The review found no strong evidence of any benefits of routine antibiotics. It also stated that not enough is known about the side-effects of antibiotics for mothers and babies. Routine antibiotics should also be avoided for the baby after birth unless there are signs of infection. In keeping with the Cochrane review, NICE guidelines recommend that: 'If there are no signs of infection, antibiotics should not be given to either the woman or the baby, even if the membranes have been ruptured for over 24 hours'.[20] Signs of infection for the mother include fever, smelly vaginal discharge and a painful uterus. Signs of infection for the baby include fever or low temperature, noisy breathing, pale skin colour and excessive sleepiness.

Women can reduce their own chance of infection after rupture of membranes by avoiding putting anything into their vagina. This includes avoiding vaginal examinations, because the more vaginal examinations a woman has, the greater her chance of getting an infection.[51] After birth, skin-to-skin contact between mother and baby allows the baby to be colonised with protective bacteria, reducing the chance of infection.[30]

My hind membranes [the part of the amniotic sac behind the baby's head] *broke along with the loss of my mucous plug at 37 weeks. I hadn't realised the occasional drips of clear fluid were actually amniotic fluid. I went in to the hospital for a check-up after six days as contractions hadn't started. Despite my baby and I being perfectly healthy and happy, the staff were alarmed and recommended I be induced on the syntocinon drip immediately, and given IV antibiotics. I didn't realise I could refuse. That option was not included in the discussion at all. What was conveyed to me was the risk to my baby and the necessity of induction (and IV antibiotics). I did ask about research at various points, and I did successfully argue to have the induction the following morning rather than immediately. Waiting gave me and my baby a chance to prepare, meditate, watch sunrise and get into a strong and clear state to birth. I also really appreciated my husband's support who, in the face of pressure from the staff, supported my decision to wait until the morning. Thanks to great birth preparation and caring midwifery support I had an incredibly joyful, smooth and empowering vaginal birth without pain medication. Now that I know more about birth I would choose to decline the induction and would run a hundred miles from the IV antibiotics.* Lana

I chose to wait out the induction as long as possible to give me the best chance of going into labour naturally. I knew statistically I was within a shot of that happening within 48 hours of my waters breaking. I didn't feel too much pressure from the medical team to be induced quicker; they seemed happy for me to wait it out, but also keen to induce. I waited about 36 hours, and made a decision for induction, but I also did it on my terms by going with the prostaglandin rather then syntocinon.   Samantha H

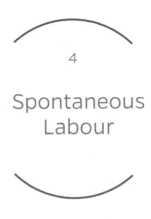

4

Spontaneous Labour

This chapter explains how a spontaneous, physiological labour works and provides a basis for understanding the induction process. A spontaneous labour is one that begins without any intervention; and the term 'physiological' refers to how a woman's body works in a healthy and natural way without the use of medicine or medical procedures. During an induction, interventions are used to produce changes in the cervix and uterus that imitate spontaneous labour. The likelihood of a successful induction is influenced by how much change has already taken place in the woman's body in preparation for labour. Oxytocin, the hormone that regulates spontaneous labour, and syntocinon, the medication used to regulate induced labour, work differently in the body. This chapter includes an explanation of how oxytocin works, and chapter 6 discusses how syntocinon alters the labour process.

How the body prepares for labour

Preparation for labour occurs throughout pregnancy, and in

particular during the final weeks. Progesterone, along with another hormone, relaxin, softens the joints in the pelvis to allow movement of the bones, creating additional space for birth. Levels of natural opiates, called beta-endorphins, begin to rise, ready to relieve the pain of labour. Both progesterone and beta-endorphins promote an inward focus and a sense of calm. Prolactin, the mothering hormone, also increases in preparation for the bonding and attachment phase following birth.

The uterus contracts regularly during pregnancy from around seven weeks. These contractions are usually pain free, and do not open the cervix. Some women are unaware of them, and other women feel them as Braxton Hicks, or 'practice' contractions. In order for the uterus to create labour contractions, changes need to occur in the uterine muscle and cervix. The hormone oxytocin is responsible for initiating and regulating the contractions of spontaneous labour. In the final weeks of pregnancy, oxytocin receptors form in the uterine muscle ready to receive and respond to increased oxytocin in the bloodstream during labour.

The cervix is the lowest part of the uterus, and holds the baby in during pregnancy. It is firm in consistency and tucked far back in the vagina, away from the pressure of the baby's head. If you have a vaginal examination in pregnancy it is likely you will be told that your cervix is 'posterior'. This is the natural place for the cervix to be during pregnancy. A firm and posterior cervix means that even when the uterus contracts, the cervix remains closed. The cervix must undergo a structural transformation to 'ripen' before it can open in response to the uterine contractions of labour. Relaxin and oestrogen initiate these structural changes and prostaglandin, leucocytes, macrophages, hyaluronic acid and glycomainoglycans are all involved in ripening the cervix. The cervix becomes softer, thinner, and moves forward to sit in front of the baby's head in an anterior position.

The cervix will ripen differently if it has opened during a previous labour. For example, it may be open at the end of pregnancy, weeks before the ripening process begins. In addition, although the cervix will soften as labour gets closer, it does not get much thinner, and can remain thick even during labour. This does not alter how well the cervix opens in labour, and usually it will open quicker than it did in a first labour once contractions are established.

Babies also undergo significant changes in the final weeks and days of pregnancy in preparation for birth, and life outside of the uterus. They lay down fat to use as energy during labour, and for their first days of establishing breastfeeding. They receive antibodies from their mother to protect them from infection and disease. As their lungs mature, surfactant is produced to enable air breathing, and fluid begins to move out of the air sacs. Their brain undergoes increased development with nerve connections being made to support breathing, temperature regulation, breastfeeding and sleeping.

Babies usually settle into a head-down position, and in first pregnancies their head may begin to move deeper into the pelvis and 'engage' into the pelvic brim. However, this is not essential, because contractions will move the baby down once labour begins. Usually the baby faces towards their mother's spine at the end of pregnancy, in an anterior position. However, many babies face outwards in a posterior position at the beginning of labour. This is a common variation, and the baby will most likely move during labour as contractions, and the shape of the pelvis encourage them to rotate to face their mother's spine.

Physiological labour

Spontaneous labour is a complex physiological process involving a number of hormones and physical changes regulated by the body, emotions and the environment.[1] The pattern of contractions, and the rate at which the cervix opens, differ enormously between individual women. While a number of hormones are involved in spontaneous labour, oxytocin plays a leading role.

Oxytocin

Oxytocin is produced primarily in the hypothalamus in the brain, and is delivered directly to the nervous system and brain. It is also transported to the pituitary gland, where it is secreted in pulses into the bloodstream, enabling it to act as a signalling substance in many areas of the body and nervous system. Oxytocin is common to all mammals and regulates the 'calm and connection' response, the opposite of the 'fight and flight' response regulated by adrenaline.[2] Oxytocin acts on the nervous system to promote relaxation and calm, and to facilitate growth and reproduction. It influences behaviours relating to bonding and connection between families, friends and sexual partners. We release oxytocin when we connect with others, for example by sharing a meal or hugging. Oxytocin is heavily involved in human reproduction and breastfeeding: it stimulates the release of eggs from the ovaries; aids in the transportation of sperm; creates uterine contractions and initiates the 'let-down' reflex for breastfeeding. It is released in high levels following orgasm and even higher levels during labour.

Early labour

What causes labour to begin is still largely unknown. The current scientific understanding suggests that the baby initiates labour by sending a hormonal signal to the mother when they are ready for external life.[3] In response, the mother's oxytocin levels rise slightly, and the oxytocin receptors in the uterine muscle become more sensitive. This combination makes uterine contractions become stronger and more noticeable. Beta-endorphins are the body's natural opiate, and they begin to rise in early labour to provide pain relief. In combination with oxytocin, beta-endorphins also encourage a calm and inward focus. However, in response to the excitement and anxiety of early labour, adrenaline is released, which activates the neocortex making the woman alert. This balance between an inward focus and alertness allows the woman to be aware of her surroundings, and organise herself and her environment for labour.

During the early phase of labour mammals, including women, seek a safe birth space, usually away from others, ready for established labour. If there is too much adrenaline, oxytocin is suppressed and contractions may stop until the balance is restored. This enables a woman in early labour to stop contracting in response to danger in the same way as other mammals do. This can be observed when a woman's contractions stop on admission to hospital and return after she has settled in and feels safe. Early labour can last many hours and sometimes days. This facilitates a steady build-up of beta-endorphins, which assist with pain relief in established labour.

Established labour
Labour is established when contractions become stronger and more powerful, and do not slow down in response to mild stress. In established labour, cortisol and beta-endorphins increase to very high levels to relieve pain and reduce stress. Beta-endorphins also help to create an altered state of

consciousness in which the woman's focus is within. Women in established labour often close their eyes and appear drowsy in between contractions due to the opiate effect of beta-endorphins. In this state neocortical functioning (the thinking part of the brain) is reduced, and the limbic system (instincts) are heightened.

Oxytocin continues to rise and, in addition to acting on the uterus, it prepares the mother and baby for the instinctive bonding behaviours that occur after birth. The mother's blood-brain barrier does not allow oxytocin to pass into it from the bloodstream. Therefore, the behavioural effects of oxytocin rely on direct delivery of oxytocin to the brain, where it is released. It also travels through the placenta via the bloodstream and passes through the much thinner blood-brain barrier of the baby. The action of the mother's oxytocin on the baby's brain during labour is believed to initiate epigenetic changes that set up the baby's own oxytocin system for life.[4]

The release of oxytocin is regulated by feedback from the baby, the uterus, the mother's emotions and the external environment. Therefore, oxytocin levels can alter during labour in response to what is going on inside the woman, and around her. This is why the birth environment is so important for labour progress. Privacy, darkness, quietness, calmness, warmth, a sense of safety, gentle touch and loving interactions promote the release of oxytocin.

Contractions and the shape of the pelvis encourage the baby to move downwards and rotate. By the end of labour most babies will be facing their mother's spine with their back against her abdomen, regardless of how they start out. A baby who starts labour with their back against their mother's spine (occipito-posterior position) will a longer rotation. A posterior position can also alter the pattern of labour, often resulting in a longer early labour phase and irregular contractions. However, once the baby's head reaches the middle of the pelvis, contractions and the round shape of the mid-pelvis create the perfect turning space. As the baby descends further, the back of the mother's pelvis (sacrum) moves up and backwards, increasing the space in the pelvis significantly. Most women instinctively take up a forward leaning position that allows the sacrum to move and gravity to assist with the downward movement of their baby.

The amniotic sac and fluid play an important role in spontaneous labour. The pressure of contractions is equalised throughout the fluid rather than directly squeezing the baby, placenta and umbilical cord. This protects the baby and their oxygen supply from the effects of uterine contractions. In addition, during contractions the amniotic fluid in front of the baby's head, called the 'forewaters', bulges downwards into the dilating cervix and eventually through into the vagina. This transmits even pressure over the cervix, helping it to open. The forewaters also protect the baby's head from direct pressure onto the cervix.

As labour progresses and birth becomes closer, there is a surge of adrenaline to counteract some of the effects of beta-endorphin. This activates the neocortex (thinking part of the brain) enough for the mother to be sufficiently alert to protect her baby immediately after birth. Some women may respond to this surge of adrenaline with sudden powerful contractions resulting in a quick birth, which is called the 'fetus ejection reflex'.[5] However, for most women this surge of adrenaline is experienced as 'transition' – a feeling of fear and overwhelm. This is a normal part of labour progress, and soon passes as the adrenaline surge clears. This is often the point at which the amniotic sac breaks as the cervix is almost fully open and the sac bulges so far into the vagina that the pressure causes it to burst. Amniotic fluid then lubricates the vagina and perineum, helping the baby to move through the vagina and stretch the perineal tissues.

Birthing the baby and placenta

Once the cervix is fully open, there may be a lull in contractions while the uterus reorganises itself around the baby as he or she moves into the vagina. As the baby descends further, pressure is applied to nerves deep in the pelvis, resulting in spontaneous pushing. Contractions become progressively expulsive as soft tissue in the perineum stretches, increasing the release of oxytocin. Oxytocin and beta-endorphin levels rise further, along with prolactin (the mothering hormone), ready to assist with the initial bonding process. The sensation of perineal tissues stretching initiates instinctive behaviours that protect the perineum from tearing. For example, the woman may hold back from pushing, gasp or scream, close her legs, and hold her perineum and the crown of her baby's head.[6] Once the baby's head is born there is likely to be a pause in contractions for a minute or so. This allows the baby time to rotate or change position to get their shoulders through the pelvis. The baby's body is usually born with the following contraction.

After the birth of the baby there is another lull in contractions as mother and baby meet each other and start interacting. During pregnancy around a third of the baby's blood is in the placenta at any one time. After birth this blood transfers into the baby via the umbilical cord. The additional circulating blood volume is mostly directed to the lungs to assist them to inflate and begin breathing. The ongoing interaction between mother and baby, and stimulation of the nipples by the baby's hands and mouth, releases further oxytocin, creating more contractions. In addition, the baby gently kicks their feet against their mother's belly as they 'crawl' to the breast, stimulating the uterus to contract. These contractions separate the placenta from the uterine wall and compress blood vessels to prevent excessive bleeding. The placenta moves through the vagina and is birthed, either with the assistance of gravity if the mother is upright, or by the woman pushing.

Spontaneous labour involves a complex interplay of hormones that influence not only labour progress, but also how the woman feels afterwards. The high levels of beta-endorphins and oxytocin circulating immediately after birth contribute to the feelings of empowerment and elation women often experience after spontaneous physiological birth.[7] There is very little research examining women's experiences of spontaneous, physiological labour. Medical intervention during labour is commonplace, and physiological birth is not the norm. The few studies that look exclusively at physiological birth identify the empowering and transformative nature of the birth experience.[8] This aspect of labour is often hidden or unacknowledged in mainstream portrayals of birth.

Women's experiences of physiological labour

Feeling how my body communicated with me was unbelievable. The way I could work with my baby on his way out was so satisfying! Also I felt protected. I was in control of everything so the pain was perfectly manageable. The power I felt for doing this huge thing, giving birth, on my own, was unbelievable. I felt like super woman. I slept, I ate, I danced, I kissed. We were in our own time. Mariana

It was the most intense and inwardly focused process of my life. Not painful (until I had to push him out!) but requiring all of me to stay with what was happening. I was amazed at how

active my mind was, thoughts racing etc. whilst appearing so tranced from the outside. The experience was so extraordinary, yet completely ordinary. I'm sad I won't ever do it again.   Jessie

My second baby was spontaneous, and her birth was the most empowering experience of my life. The contractions gradually built up, there's no denying that they hurt but it was manageable. I think because the pain was manageable I was able to focus on my body and my baby. I felt clarity within myself and, as clichéd as it sounds, my body knew what to do. It reframed my perspective around the birthing process that had been very tainted from my first labour. Although I understand there are certain situations where it's not an option, it's a feeling that every woman deserves to feel. It's liberating!   Meg

Normal birth feels big. Everything feels big inside, and the world outside shrinks. The early period pain sensations strengthen to waves that need to be ridden. Unlike some women, I do find it painful; there's no escaping that reality. The bigness of everything can be overwhelming. The sensation builds and I need to release it through my mouth, with my voice. I groan, I vocalise, I 'ahhhhh', I 'AHHHHH', and I roar. And then, I grunt and bear down (usually after I've had a meltdown of some variety; not wanting to accept that there's more work to be done and not realising how much work has already been done). It is all consuming and nothing else matters. Except making sure everyone else is quiet. I'm the noisy one, and no one else can be. I'm so self-absorbed, unapologetically so. And when I feel baby moving down, it's the best feeling knowing you're almost there. The ring of fire is real, the birth of the head is incredible, and that last push as baby is born is the absolute best. All the relief. All the joy. Is there a word for relief-joy? There should be. And your fresh newborn is in your arms, taking his or her first breath, and that's another level of relief-joy. And you take a moment to breathe, and look at your baby's sex. And then you realise there's the placenta left to birth. It's not over yet. So you get that done and THEN you can relax.   *Anna*

Trusting in my body, and allowing myself the time to do what is so physiologically normal was one of the most life-changing experiences of my life. It changed how I viewed myself as a woman, and as a mother. It forever empowered me and set a fire within my soul that meant I can do anything. It forever changed me, and to it I am forever grateful as a woman.   *Jessica*

All four of my labours were spontaneous, and although they each began differently, I found myself surrendering my body and self to the process of birth once labour began (why try and control what can't be controlled?). I was calm, focused and went within myself with each birth, and was able to ride the surges with no need for pain relief. I was well supported through each delivery with wonderful midwives who were hands off, but still very supportive and encouraging, and they allowed me the space I needed to deliver my babies myself, in my own time. I found all of my labours and births to be so empowering and amazing. I felt so strong and capable of anything after each of them. I am forever in awe of what my body is capable of. Physiological birth is simply wonderful.   *Rebecca*

I woke up at about 6.30am and rolled to the side to go to the bathroom and felt pop, yep my membranes had ruptured. Throughout the day I had no regularity to contractions but at about 1pm I explained to my husband that things were happening and baby would be born that day. We found time together and just let the labour build. Ahh it was beautiful, enjoying the intensity getting stronger, as the stronger it got, the closer I knew I was to meeting our baby. That moment of needing to be in the room I would give birth in. The moment of getting into the pool and knowing I was ready to have my baby. The moment of birth. Often I still close my eyes and remember the feelings of my birth – I could do it all again any day, it was perfect.   Alice

My second birth, a VBAC [vaginal birth after caesarean], was a long and slow labour and I was wrecked. But as soon as my baby was in my arms and for the rest of that day, I was absolutely buzzing! I literally felt like I could do anything in the world. Like I could have conquered Mount Everest. I felt invincible. I felt incredible. And because of how I battled to get my VBAC, and to be left alone, I felt like a bit of a hero because all the midwives were backing me secretly and the obstetricians were hating me. So afterwards, all the midwives I saw were so happy and grinning for me.   Kimberley

I had one completely spontaneous labour and birth with no intervention. This was the most beautiful and empowering moment in my life. To bring my baby into the world, trusting myself and my body to allow me to do so on my terms, was the most defining moment in my womanhood.   Samantha D

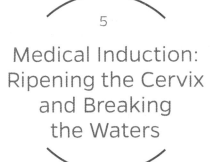

5

Medical Induction: Ripening the Cervix and Breaking the Waters

There are three steps in an induction process: ripening the cervix; breaking the amniotic sac (the waters) and creating contractions. The first two steps are aimed at preparing the body to respond effectively to induced contractions. The cervix needs to ripen and change in structure so that it can open with labour contractions. The first step of the induction process involves using interventions to produce changes in the cervix. The amount of intervention needed depends on a number of factors, in particular how close the woman is to spontaneous labour. Some women will go into labour in response to the interventions used to ripen the cervix, or after their water has been broken. However, most women, in particular those having their first baby, will require a syntocinon drip to create labour contractions.

Assessing the cervix

Before starting the induction process, an assessment of the cervix is carried out to help plan the most appropriate method of induction. The cervix is assessed during a vaginal examination, and evaluated by scoring a number of factors. The overall score is called the 'Bishop score', and the higher the score, the more 'favourable' to induction the cervix is considered to be. The most common form of the Bishop score is the modified version, which assesses:

- Dilation: how open the cervix is
- Effacement: whether the cervix is thick or thin
- Station: how low the cervix is in the pelvis
- Consistency: how soft the cervix is
- Position: whether the opening is posterior or anterior

The Bishop score is not a very accurate way of predicting how successful induction will be.[1] However, the findings can be used to inform the next step in the induction process. For example, if the Bishop score is high, there may be no need for interventions aimed at ripening the cervix.

Ripening the cervix

If the Bishop score is low, the next step in the induction process is to ripen the cervix so that it will open with labour contractions. The other reason for ripening the cervix is to open it enough to break the amniotic sac, which is the following step in the induction process (see below). Although a number of hormones are involved in naturally ripening the cervix, prostaglandins are the focus in the induction process. All the interventions aimed at ripening the cervix attempt to either release the body's own prostaglandins, or to introduce synthetic prostaglandins. Prostaglandins are part of the body's natural inflammatory response. They are responsible for increasing the blood flow to a damaged area, and summoning white blood cells that protect the body against infection. The action of prostaglandins can be seen when a red raised mark develops in response to a scratch on the skin. Prostaglandins act on the cervix to increase blood flow, encouraging the tissues to soften and stretch. In some cases, when a woman is close to labour herself, procedures aimed at ripening the cervix might initiate spontaneous labour without the need for further interventions. There are a number of methods used to ripen the cervix: membrane sweeping, pharmaceutical prostaglandins and mechanical devices.

Membrane sweeping
A membrane sweep, or 'stretch and sweep' is usually the first intervention used to stimulate prostaglandin release in the cervix. This intervention is often offered towards the end of pregnancy in an attempt to reduce the chance of post-dates pregnancy. However, a membrane sweep is a form of induction because it is an intervention that aims to make the body go into labour before labour would have happened naturally.

A membrane sweep involves a vaginal examination in which the midwife or doctor puts a finger into the cervical opening and sweeps it around inside the cervix in an attempt to separate the amniotic sac from the lower part of the uterus. If they are unable to get their finger into the cervix, the outside of the cervix will be swept instead. A membrane sweep causes irritation to the cervix and lower uterus, which releases prostaglandins. The procedure is not gentle, and a certain amount of discomfort is required to stimulate prostaglandin release and make the intervention effective. Common side-effects of this procedure include pain, bleeding from the cervix and irregular contractions.[2] If the cervix is open at the time of the procedure there is a risk of accidentally rupturing the amniotic sac.[3] In some cases, a membrane sweep causes a prolonged pre-labour phase in which the woman can experience painful contractions for days without getting into established labour. This can be exhausting and frustrating, and often results in the need for an epidural and further interventions.

The effectiveness of a membrane sweep is difficult to evaluate because it is impossible to know which women were about to go into spontaneous labour regardless of the intervention. For example, many women will go into labour the day after their membrane sweep, but they may have done that anyway without the membrane sweep. A Cochrane review of the research into this procedure found that it reduced the need for further induction interventions for one in eight women.[2] Most of the studies included in the review involved multiple membrane sweeps: weekly or in some cases every 48 hours from 38 weeks onwards. The review concluded that membrane sweeping does 'not seem to produce clinically important benefits' when used to prevent the need for further induction interventions. Therefore, the value of routine membrane sweeping to avoid further induction interventions is debatable. However, the procedure makes sense as a first step in the induction process once a woman has decided to undergo induction, and it can be carried out during the Bishop score assessment (see above).

I had two membrane sweeps with my induction. One was three days before my induction, and the second one was done when they did my ARM [artificial rupture of membranes]. Having a membrane sweep when your cervix is posterior, long and closed, or only slightly open is incredibly uncomfortable. There is an intense pressure that takes your breath away while the procedure is being done, but as soon as it's over, the pressure subsides. For me, the membrane sweep started some back pain and very mild tightening. My mucous plug came away, and my cervix changed from 1cm dilated and 2cm long, to 3cm dilated and 1cm long, which made the ARM easier.   Samantha L

My first membrane sweep was at 37 weeks. It was extremely uncomfortable and I had a small amount of blood afterwards. Nothing came of it. I had my second at 38 weeks, but baby pulled his head away so it was a failed attempt. They tried again at 39 weeks, with more blood than the first time, but yet again nothing came from it. I didn't go into labour at all.   Tiara

I had a membrane sweep at 38+4 weeks. It was uncomfortable in the sense that someone had their fingers inside me, but I wouldn't say it hurt. Within one hour I began having contractions. I thought it was just from the sweep so carried on until I noticed they were quite regular. I was having contractions every 3–4 minutes. After a few hours I decided to go into hospital as I was scared of having an unplanned home birth. Once I arrived at hospital things began to slow down. I was checked after a few hours, and there was no change to my cervix from when I had the sweep, so we went home. Contractions continued during the rest of the night until morning came and they stopped. After a small sleep at midday they started again and baby was born that evening.   Jade

With my first I had several membrane sweeps. I now understand they are a form of induction, and one of the risks is a prolonged pre-labour. I had about 10 days of stop-start labour, which I think was partly due to the sweeps. Arianwen

Pharmaceutical ripening
If a membrane sweep does not initiate labour, or sufficiently ripen the cervix, the next step for most women is to apply

synthetic prostaglandins near the cervix. There are a number of manufacturers of prostaglandins, so the medication has different trade names, including dinoprost, cervidil and prostin E2. Each medication package includes a 'patient information leaflet', which should be given to the woman receiving the medication. The leaflet includes information about the dosage, administration, side-effects and risks.

Prostaglandins are inserted high in the vagina next to the cervix during a vaginal examination. The medication may be in the form of a gel, or a pessary with a tape that hangs out of the vagina. The dosage of prostaglandin used will depend on the woman's individual circumstances. For example, lower doses are usually used for women who have laboured in a previous pregnancy. Occasionally, prostaglandins are given as an oral tablet (misoprostol) rather than vaginally. Prostaglandins will be administered in a hospital setting because the woman and baby need to be monitored closely. For the woman, this will involve having her blood pressure, pulse, breathing rate and any uterine contractions monitored over at least a four-hour period. The baby's heart rate will be assessed using a CTG (continuous cardiotocograph) machine for at least 30 minutes, and then regularly with a Doppler for at least four hours after administration.

Usually, once the process of artificially ripening the cervix has begun, the woman will remain in hospital until the baby is born. The cervix will be reassessed a number of hours after the administration of prostaglandin – 6 after gel, and 12 after a pessary. If there has been no change, or little change, another dose of prostaglandin will be given or a mechanical method of ripening used instead (see below). If the cervix has opened enough, the woman will move onto the next step in the induction process: breaking the amniotic sac.

It is common to experience sharp pains around the

cervix and uncomfortable uterine cramps in response to prostaglandins. Care providers often refer to this discomfort as 'prostin pains'. Less common side-effects include nausea, vomiting, diarrhoea and fever.[4] Rarely, prostaglandins cause hyperstimulation of the uterus, resulting in excessive contractions which can be dangerous for mother and baby. If there are signs of hyperstimulation, attempts will be made to remove the prostaglandin, by either washing it out in the case of gel, or pulling it out in the case of a pessary. If the hyperstimulation continues, an emergency caesarean may be necessary to deliver the baby quickly.

I had my first baby 5 months ago. I opted for the prostin as I was willing to try anything to avoid the ARM and syntocinon. I had done lots of acupuncture and membrane sweeps in the week prior and was 3cm dilated without any contractions. After the prostin went in, it was all on! The insertion itself wasn't any more painful than a sweep (probably less painful for me actually). Baby coped fine with it, and within a few minutes I had my first contraction. They didn't stop after that! It took about five hours for the contractions to get very painful and to establish labour. I was lucky to have a very experienced private midwife, and even though I birthed in a hospital, I opted for a water birth (often not allowed in hospital after prostin). We had a beautiful birth less than 10 hours after the prostin went in. I had a great outcome! Katrina

Prostin gel, to me, feels like a very stingy period pain. It made my upper thighs burn, and my cervix ache. It made my cervix soft enough to be able to proceed with an ARM, but it did not send me into labour. It was the first step of many. My labours that have not involved prostin gel start off way more pleasant, and I don't feel as irritable. Lynda

My waters broke dead on 37 weeks around 6pm. Just a trickle. After another day and night and no signs of any labour I agreed to be induced by prostaglandins first. The pessary was put in and I was given a sweep without permission and told I was 1cm. I quickly went into hyperstimulation and the pessary was removed. Things calmed down and I was able to keep baby calm too as she had been in distress and she did pass some meconium. But I managed to keep baby calm by staying calm myself.   Sam Hatton

This was my second birth so I have something to compare it to. With my first I went into labour naturally. With my second I had prostin gel applied, and after the first dose had a few cramps. After the second dose was applied I went into labour so there was no need for the drip. I had lots of burning and stinging sensations in my cervix after both doses of prostin, but after the second dose, cramping turned into labour. The labour was much more intense and very painful compared to my natural birth previously. It seemed like the pain was excruciating right from the start when I was only 2cm dilated. With my first baby I slept through the initial stages of early labour, and only got to the hospital when I was 4cm dilated. With the second, after the prostin, at 4cm I was already asking for an epidural.   Kasia

It was a quite uncomfortable procedure getting the prostin applied. Within around five minutes of insertion I had quite a strong reaction and had a tonic [excessive and prolonged] contraction which caused my baby to become quite distressed. This was the trigger for the emergency c-section under full general anaesthetic. It was very traumatic to experience this as it wasn't discussed with me as a potential reaction to the procedure or drug. Reflecting on it since then, I think they only pushed me

into the prostin gel path to be actively trying to do something
instead of just waiting to see how things went.   *Hayley*

Mechanical ripening

The mechanical method of cervical ripening relies on the woman's own production of prostaglandins. This method is often recommended for women who have an increased chance of hyperstimulation with pharmaceutical prostaglandins. It may also be used if the pharmaceutical method does not work effectively. The mechanical method involves placing an inflatable balloon or double balloon into the lower part of the uterus to sit between the amniotic sac and the cervix. The balloon is passed through the cervix uninflated on the end of a rubber tube, then inflated with 30–80mls of sterile solution so that it is unable to pass back through the cervix. Traction may be applied to the balloon by taping the tubing to the woman's leg. By applying constant pressure on the cervix the balloon stimulates the release of prostaglandins. It also stretches the cervix, which may encourage oxytocin release and stimulate contractions. The balloon will fall out once it has stretched the cervix enough to escape. When this occurs the amniotic sac is broken quickly before the cervix closes again (see below). If the balloon does not fall out, the cervix will be reassessed after 12 hours of the device being inserted.

Common side-effects of having a balloon device inserted include discomfort and cramping. However, women report less discomfort with mechanical methods of cervical ripening than with pharmaceutical methods.[5] Occasionally, the amniotic sac is accidentally ruptured during the procedure, but this is the next step in the induction process anyway. The balloon can also push the baby upwards out of the pelvis. This makes breaking the waters more risky, because it increases the chance that the baby's umbilical cord can get in front of the baby's head. The baby may also move into a position that requires a caesarean, for example, lying across the uterus. Rarely, the balloon device becomes trapped in the cervix, making it difficult to remove.

I had the balloon catheter the night before my son's birth. I had cramping, the same as if I was having bad period pain. I used a heat pack, but still managed to get some sleep. I woke at 7am, went to the toilet, and the balloon had fallen out successfully. There was a decent sized blood clot attached to the balloon. At 7:30am my waters were broken. Hayley Jean

I had the balloon catheter inserted after one failed attempt with prostin. My cervix was very sore by the time the balloon was inserted. I could only take 60ml of water in the balloon, as I was sore and bleeding after insertion. I was also having contractions at the time they were inserting it. Afterwards I started to get period-type cramps and my contractions became more painful. I ended up taking pain relief and a sleeping tablet to get some sleep. Some time early the next morning my contractions stopped all together and they had to take it out as it did not fall out itself. It didn't make me go into labour. Sam

I had a balloon catheter after the prostin gel didn't work. Everything about it was incredibly painful. Putting it in was painful, and actually quite humiliating. After it was in, I went into the toilet to get some time out, and I just started throwing up (I think maybe my body was in shock). A short time after that I started getting cramps unlike anything I've ever had, and I had to have pethidine to stop the pain. I didn't find this 'thing' dangling in my pants too bad, and it was uncomfortable when it was taken out, but not too bad. I tried to research induction methods before I was induced, and I think I read that this method is the preferred method in my local hospital. I can't believe this horrible method is the preferred means of induction!   *Linda*

Breaking the amniotic sac

Breaking the amniotic sac to release the fluid from around the baby is the next step in the induction process.[*] This is called 'artificial rupture of membranes' and is often referred to by its acronym, 'ARM'. An ARM is sometimes carried out during a spontaneous labour in an attempt to speed up the labour. However, it does not speed up spontaneous labour, and can result in unnecessary complications.[6] In contrast, during an induced labour, fluid around the baby can prevent induced contractions from getting into an effective pattern. So, unlike in a spontaneous labour, breaking the amniotic sac makes an induced labour quicker.[7] In addition, an ARM may reduce the chance of an amniotic fluid embolism occurring during induction. An amniotic fluid embolism is an extremely rare complication (6 per 100,000 births), and one cause is thought to be induced contractions forcing amniotic fluid through the placenta into the bloodstream and into the woman's lungs.[8] An ARM removes the amniotic fluid, thereby reducing the chance of this very rare complication.

The amniotic sac is broken using an amnihook, which is a device that looks like a long crochet hook. The amnihook is introduced into the vagina and through the opening of the cervix, where it is used to tear a hole in the part of the amniotic sac that sits just inside the cervix. The midwife or doctor then uses their finger to make the hole in the sac bigger until amniotic fluid is released. There are no nerve endings in the amniotic sac, so tearing the sac is not painful. However,

---

[*] In the United States this is not always part of the induction process.

the procedure can be uncomfortable because the amnihook is moved around inside the vagina and cervix. Research also suggests that the baby has an initial stress response to the amniotic sac being broken.[9] This may result in the baby's heartrate increasing for a minute or so after the procedure.

There are some risks associated with the ARM procedure. The cervix may bleed if it is bumped or nicked with the amnihook. Occasionally, the baby's head is scratched by the amnihook, particularly if the amniotic sac is tight over the baby's head. Once the protective amniotic sac is broken there is an increased chance of infection, particularly if a number of vaginal examinations are carried out afterwards. There are also some rare complications associated with ARM. If a blood vessel from the placenta is running through the amniotic sac (velamentous insertion of the umbilical cord), it can be accidentally punctured with the amnihook, resulting in bleeding from the baby and placenta. The umbilical cord can be washed out of the uterus with the amniotic fluid (cord prolapse) if the baby's head is not firmly settled in the pelvis. Both of these complications require an emergency caesarean to deliver the baby.

For some women, an ARM itself will result in spontaneous uterine contractions and labour will start without the need for further intervention. Therefore, some women choose to wait and see what happens for an hour or more after their ARM. If spontaneous contractions do begin, the labour is still considered induced, and will be treated as an induced labour in terms of increased monitoring of wellbeing and progress, particularly if the cervix was ripened using pharmaceutical prostaglandin.

With my second baby, I had an ARM. It was a strange moment – I remember feeling thankful my cervix was dilated and the midwife could break my waters. The midwife was so kind, and had my consent, and talked it through gently. It was a feeling of relief when the waters went – weirdly I remember liking the feeling (gosh I sound strange)! Then the midwife said 'there is no way you are having syntocinon', and she cranked up the radio and said 'dance this baby out!' She said I had two hours to get into established labour. Two and a half hours later she said 'you are in good enough labour for me' – no vaginal examination. Then thirty minutes later Erin was born – all fours on the bed, still with the terrible Magic radio on!   Alice

I had my waters broken via ARM for my first baby. The actual procedure didn't worry me at the time, somewhat similar to a pap smear, but it ended with me sitting in a puddle of mess, which I guess is a bit weird in hindsight. Straight away I started to feel some contractions that were building so I was excited, and I believed this was the closest I was going to get to a natural labour. It was the interventions that followed (syntocinon drip then eventually forceps) that made my labour forced, artificial and far too quick (5.5 hours in total). I often wonder what my body could have done if we had allowed it to continue to labour after the ARM. Given there were no imminent medical risks to myself or the baby, I'm not sure why everyone was in such a rush. I also think I would have seen induction as a positive experience had no further interventions been introduced. Meg

I had an ARM as part of my induction process for my first baby. I was 2cm dilated and it wasn't painful (although it was more than 24 hours after the last round of prostin, which probably helped). No risks were discussed with me at all. The procedure itself was quite uncomfortable, and not very pleasant, as much as the midwife tried to be gentle. It was a very odd sensation, with the water leaking out underneath me. I was wearing pads so that I could keep mobile and moving. Every time I moved another huge gush would come out. I also had some blood on the pad. I stated at the time that I didn't want any syntocinon, but they still put in a cannula and set a drip up. I assume it was saline, but I never actually asked, nor was it discussed. I assumed this was normal, and didn't question it all. I had fairly regular contractions pretty quickly afterwards, but not quickly enough for the obstetrician on duty. At that stage, I didn't understand that broken waters put me on the clock.   Helen

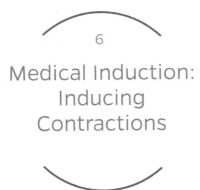

6

Medical Induction: Inducing Contractions

Once the cervix is ripe and the amniotic fluid is removed, the next step in the induction process is to create labour contractions. An induced labour aims to open the cervix by creating contractions with a synthetic version of oxytocin. However, induction does not involve the other hormones in the same way as spontaneous labour (see chapter 4). In addition, early labour is bypassed, making an induced labour generally quicker than a spontaneous labour, once contractions are established.

Syntocinon

Induced contractions are created using a medication called syntocinon, an artificial form of oxytocin (known as pitocin in the United States). The chemical make-up of syntocinon is exactly the same as oxytocin, and it acts on oxytocin receptors in the uterine muscle in the same way. However, there are some important differences in the way syntocinon functions. Firstly, syntocinon is administered directly into the bloodstream at a

Oxytocin	Syntocinon
Released in pulses from the mother's brain and is influenced by feedback from the baby, the uterus, the mother's emotions, and the birth environment.	Released at a constant rate into the blood stream via a drip, and the rate is unaffected by other factors.
Acts on the mother's brain in addition to the uterus.	Unable to cross the mother's blood-brain barrier and acts only on the uterus.
Crosses the blood-brain barrier of the baby in small volumes.	Can cross the blood-brain barrier of the baby in very high volumes.

Table 1: Key differences between oxytocin and syntocinon.

constant rate via an intravenous drip, and therefore cannot be altered by feedback from the baby, the uterus, the woman's emotions or the environment. Secondly, it is unable to pass through the mother's blood-brain barrier to reach her brain. Syntocinon in the bloodstream also reduces the release of oxytocin in the brain. Therefore, unlike oxytocin, syntocinon is unable to influence the mother's bonding behaviours. Thirdly, it can cross the thin blood-brain barrier of the baby in larger quantities than oxytocin. This may alter the baby's oxytocin system and bonding behaviours such as eye contact and sucking at the breast.[1]

Syntocinon-induced contractions
During an induced labour, an intravenous cannula is inserted into a vein, and a drip containing syntocinon is started. The

rate of this drip starts very slow, because every woman responds differently to the medication. Some women may only need a very small amount of syntocinon to have strong contractions, while others may need a lot. The rate is increased every half an hour until the uterus is contracting about three to four times every ten minutes. The frequency of contractions is measured in 10-minute intervals, and care providers use the terminology 3:10 or 4:10. The drip then continues until after the baby is born. One small study tested what happened when syntocinon was stopped after the women's contraction pattern was established.[2] Around half of the women in the study needed to have the syntocinon started again. However, the other half were able to continue their labour without syntocinon.

The pain experienced during induced contractions is different from the pain of spontaneous labour for a number of reasons. The induction process skips early labour, with strong contractions usually occurring within two hours of starting the syntocinon drip. This does not allow time for the woman's body to slowly and steadily raise beta-endorphin levels to relieve pain. The brain is also not releasing oxytocin to help create a sense of calm. In addition, induced contractions are kept at a strong and steady rate once they are in an effective pattern. They do not alter and provide periods of rest or reduced intensity like in spontaneous labour. Not surprisingly, women undergoing induction have an increased chance of requiring pain relief, especially those having their first labour induced.[3]

There are a number of additional interventions required during an induced labour. There will be a cannula (IV) placed in the hand or arm, attached to the drip of syntocinon. The baby's heart rate and the contraction pattern will be monitored continuously using a cardiotocograph (CTG) machine. This involves having two sensors strapped to the abdomen and attached to a machine to generate a recording of how the baby is responding to contractions. The drip and CTG monitor will reduce the ability to move to some extent, and will usually prevent the woman from using the shower or the bath. However, there are CTG monitors that use telemetry rather than cables to communicate the information from the sensors to the recording machine, and some that have waterproof sensors. These monitors allow women to move more freely and use water during labour. However, waterbirth is not recommended during an induced labour due to the possible effects of syntocinon on the baby (see below). The effectiveness of contractions will be assessed by regular vaginal examinations. While vaginal examinations are not recommended as a means of determining progress in a spontaneous labour,[4] in an induction it is important to ensure that the induced contractions are opening the cervix.

After the birth of the baby, additional syntocinon will be given either via the cannula, or as an injection into the thigh. This is called 'active management' of the placenta, and may also involve the care provider pulling on the umbilical cord to remove the placenta (see chapter 8 for options regarding active management). Active management is recommended after an induced labour because the woman will not release the post-birth burst of oxytocin that occurs in a spontaneous labour. Without active management there is an increased chance of losing more blood than normal after birth (post-partum haemorrhage).

Occasionally syntocinon fails to create effective labour contractions, and the induction process does not progress. This may occur because the oxytocin receptors in the uterine muscle have not had enough time to develop in late pregnancy (see Chapter 4). If this happens, the next step will depend on the individual situation. Further attempts at cervical ripening

Intervention	Reason for intervention
Intravenous cannula – a drip placed in the vein of a hand, wrist or arm	To administer syntocinon and any other medications required during the induction process
Regular vaginal examinations – at least four-hourly	To ensure that the induced contractions are opening the cervix effectively
Continuous cardiotocograph (CTG) monitoring of the contraction pattern and baby's heart rate	To identify hyperstimulation of the uterus, and assess how well the baby is coping with induced contractions
Active management of the placenta – administration of a high dose of syntocinon, and traction on the umbilical cord to deliver the placenta	To mimic the burst of post-birth oxytocin that occurs in spontaneous labour and to reduce the chance of excessive bleeding

Table 2: Additional interventions required during an induced labour

may be tried before recommencing syntocinon. In some cases, the recommendation may be to go home for 24 hours, then start the process again. However, usually, once the decision has been made to deliver the baby, the process continues until the baby is born. A caesarean is often recommended following an unsuccessful induction.

I had heard lots of stories that syntocinon makes contractions unbearably painful, but my memory of labour was that it was not too bad with just gas and air, although the contractions did take my breath away right at the end. However, there was one incident when the contractions were right on top of each other, and my dose was dropped back a bit. I think it was a bit scary for my mum who was with me, and the midwife rushed off to call the obstetrician. I had a vaginal birth with vacuum assistance. I don't believe I was fully informed that I would be given syntocinon straight away after my waters were broken. I was actually really disappointed when I realised I was going to be tied to a drip, I couldn't have a shower, and I couldn't walk around. Consequently it also put focus on the bed as the appropriate place to labour, and I couldn't do other things like just get things from my bag (like food). It really forced me to be passive in my labour and in my presence in the room generally.   *Linda*

The moment the drip went in it was as though I had been whacked in the stomach with a sledge hammer... again and again and again! There was very little, if any, time between contractions, and I'm pretty sure at one stage my head spun around like something out of The Exorcist. *I felt the urge to bear down with every contraction, and spent half my labour on the toilet... not exactly the natural water birth I had been dreaming of for nine months. It was out of control and simply horrible. I opted for no pain relief but used a TENS machine. My baby was born vaginally with forceps as I was given strict time frames and apparently I was taking too long. I can still feel those forceps!*   *Meg*

I had syntocinon with my third baby after two spontaneous labours. It was tough – nothing prepared me for the pain that comes with it. It is forcing your body to do something it's not ready for! My midwife was fantastic and as soon as I was contracting effectively the syntocinon was turned off.   Tracey

I avoided analgesics during the induction, instead opting to use the shower, a fit ball and the TENS machine I had hired. However, it was a largely uncomfortable experience on the whole. In addition to the simulated 'contractions', there was also the cannula in my hand, the limited mobility due to monitoring, and the discomfort of the CTG belts around my belly.   *Tessa*

Side-effects and complications

Induction of labour should only be carried out because there are concerns for the wellbeing of the mother and/or baby if the pregnancy continues. Therefore, any potential complications of induction need to be weighed against the risks of continuing the pregnancy. Chapters 2 and 3 discuss common situations in which induction is recommended, and Chapter 1 provides guidance for making decisions about induction.

Most of the side-effects and complications discussed below are general to the use of syntocinon in labour. However, women having their first labour induced have a different set of risks in comparison to women having a subsequent labour induced: these differences will be identified where relevant. Most of the complications associated with induction can be lessened and/ or managed using further intervention. It is also important to remember that while most women will experience some side-effects of induction, most do not encounter any of the rare complications.

Hyperstimulation

A common side-effect of syntocinon is hyperstimulation of the uterus.[3] Any contraction, induced or spontaneous, compresses the placenta causing a temporary reduction in blood flow and oxygen to the baby. Blood flow through the placenta resumes when the uterus relaxes between contractions. These normal interruptions to the oxygen supply of the baby initiate physiological changes that prepare the baby for breathing after birth. Babies who do not experience labour contractions, like those born by elective caesarean, are more likely to have problems establishing breathing at birth.[5]

Hyperstimulation occurs because a contraction pattern regulated by syntocinon cannot respond to feedback from the baby or uterus. Unlike spontaneous contractions, induced contractions can be too strong, too close together, or last for too long. In addition, during an induction, the baby does not have the protection of the amniotic fluid to help diffuse the pressure of a contraction. Instead, contractions directly compress the placenta, the baby, and often the umbilical cord. Without enough time between contractions for the uterus to relax sufficiently to replenish the oxygen supply, the baby will become stressed. Hyperstimulation can be identified by closely monitoring the contraction pattern and the baby's heart rate with a CTG machine. If hyperstimulation occurs, the syntocinon infusion can be turned down or off, which will reduce the contractions and usually alleviate the problem.

If hyperstimulation is not managed it can become dangerous for the baby. In rare cases, excessive contractions can cause the placenta to detach from the uterine wall (abruption), or the uterine muscle can tear (uterine rupture). However, a more common scenario is the inability to create strong enough contractions to make the cervix open at the same time as avoiding hyperstimulation. Either the labour does not progress, or the baby becomes distressed. This is the most common reason for an induction of labour ending in a caesarean.

Caesarean
There is some debate about whether induction of labour increases a woman's chance of a having a caesarean. Most research on this topic is about the management of post-dates

pregnancy in a general population. These studies combine the outcomes for women having their first baby with those having subsequent babies, and report that induction does not increase the chance of caesarean. However, an Australian study examining birth outcomes for women having their first baby after an uncomplicated pregnancy found that induction more than doubled the chance of an emergency caesarean. The caesarean rate was 12.5% for women in spontaneous labour compared to 26.5% for women being induced.[6] Another study carried out in the UK found an even higher rate of caesarean for women having their first labour induced: 39.9% compared to 17.5% of women in spontaneous labour.[3] This study looked at births between 2007 and 2008, so the rates are likely to be higher for both groups now due to the general increase in caesareans over the years. The reason for an increased rate of caesarean for women having their first baby has not been researched. It may be that first labours tend to be longer, and this means the baby is subjected to syntocinon-induced contractions for a longer period of time. In addition, higher doses of syntocinon are usually required in a first labour. Women who have laboured before tend to respond very quickly to syntocinon. Therefore, it is easier to create effective contractions with much lower doses of syntocinon. The combination of lower doses of syntocinon, and less time in labour, may reduce the chance of the baby becoming distressed.

Malposition of the baby and shoulder dystocia
During a spontaneous labour the baby moves and adjusts their position when the uterus is relaxed between contractions. In particular, at the end of labour when the baby is being pushed out, contractions space out, allowing the baby time to rotate their shoulders to fit through the pelvis. Induced contractions

tend to be more consistent and frequent, and may not provide as much opportunity for movement in between contractions. Therefore, the baby is more likely to get into a difficult position during an induced labour, causing problems with moving through the pelvis.[7] If the baby is unable to rotate their shoulders through the pelvis after their head is born, they may get stuck (shoulder dystocia), which requires emergency management.

Perineal tearing
In a spontaneous labour, the birth of the baby through the vagina is fairly slow, providing time for the perineal tissues to stretch. However, syntocinon can make this phase of labour quicker, in particular for women who have previously had a vaginal birth. This faster birth increases the chance of perineal tearing.[8]

Neonatal complications at birth
An induced labour, and in particular the induction of a first labour, increases the chance that the baby will require resuscitation at birth.[3] Even when other factors are taken into account, such as the reason for induction, the use of syntocinon in labour is associated with an increased chance of cerebral palsy.[9] These outcomes are probably due to the effects of unmanaged hyperstimulation described above. Complications may also be related to the difference in pushing contractions at the end of an induced labour. In a spontaneous labour, contractions usually slow down during the pushing phase, allowing the baby more recovery time between contractions. This helps the baby to cope with the additional head compression, and reduction in blood flow that occurs as they move through the vagina. Induced contractions do not space out at the end of labour to provide this additional recovery time.

Post-partum haemorrhage

There is an increased chance of a post-partum haemorrhage (excessive bleeding) following an induced labour. If the oxytocin receptors on the uterus become saturated with syntocinon they are unable to respond to further syntocinon. If this happens, the additional dose of syntocinon given to actively manage the placenta will be ineffective. Therefore, after the placenta has separated from the wall of the uterus there are inadequate contractions to compress the exposed blood vessels and stop bleeding.[10] If a post-partum haemorrhage occurs, other medications and methods will be used to make the uterus contract.

Water retention

Syntocinon encourages water retention in both mother and baby. For the mother this may be seen as increased oedema or a swollen cervix. In extremely rare cases it can lead to water intoxication. For the baby, water retention results in a higher birth weight due to the additional weight of fluid. The baby will pass the additional fluid through urination in the first days after birth. However, this is important to take into consideration when weighing the baby during the first week after birth. The baby may incorrectly appear to have lost excessive weight in comparison to their birth weight. This can lead to unnecessary recommendations about feeding, and delayed discharge home based on misguided concerns about the baby's weight loss.

Difficulty with establishing breastfeeding

Women who have syntocinon during labour are three times less likely to initiate breastfeeding in the first four hours after birth; are twice as likely to give formula to their baby in hospital,[11] and have reduced rates of breastfeeding at two months.[1] Prolactin is the hormone that regulates breastmilk production, and oxytocin initiates the release of milk from the breast. Both of these hormones rely on stimulation of the breast and removal of breastmilk. In particular, the first hours and days of breastfeeding are important for establishing the future potential breastmilk supply. Michel Odent suggests three reasons for the association between syntocinon and difficulties with breastfeeding.[1] Firstly, high concentrations of syntocinon may de-sensitise the oxytocin receptors in the breast. Secondly, high concentrations of syntocinon may alter the maternal oxytocin system via a feedback mechanism that weakens the mother's hormonal response to suckling. Thirdly, high levels of syntocinon in the baby's brain may alter the behaviour of the baby, and studies have linked syntocinon in labour to diminished feeding behaviours in babies.[11]

Maternal depression and anxiety

The use of syntocinon in labour has been linked to an increased chance of depression and anxiety disorders in the first year after birth.[12] This may be related to the effects of syntocinon on the mother's oxytocin system. However, this link may also be associated with factors that are more likely to occur if labour is induced, for example, intervention during birth and/or difficulty with breastfeeding.

Behavioural disorders in childhood

Labour is thought to initiate epigenetic changes that set the oxytocin system for the baby.[13] Syntocinon can pass through the baby's blood-brain barrier in larger volumes than oxytocin, and this may alter the set point of the baby's oxytocin system long term. Research suggests there is a link between the use of syntocinon for induction and the development of autism, and attention deficit hyperactivity disorder (ADHD).[14,15]

However, at present this is only an association, rather than a confirmation of causation, and there are likely to be many other causes of ADHD and autism.

I agreed to syntocinon two hours after I had my waters broken. The risks were not explained to me. At first it didn't feel any different to the contractions I was already having, but once it was up to a 4, I was having very, very intense contractions without a break. At this point (also while my Midwifery Group Practice midwife was out of the room) I asked for the epidural. While waiting for the epidural, I asked them to turn the syntocinon drip down, which they did, and I found contractions to once again be bearable. I still went ahead with the epidural, because at this stage I was very scared of the pain ahead and had just had an internal and been told I was 4cm. I progressed to fully dilated and after two hours of pushing was taken for a c-section for failure to progress, due to a malpositioned baby. Helen

This was my first labour and I felt completely in control and was managing fine. The syntocinon went in when I was 7cm with no progress within their time frames. Once it was in, my contractions went from manageable to unbearable. I had been coping on my own fine without any pain relief. Within the hour contractions were on top of each other, with no break in between, and I made the request for an epidural. As we prepped for the epidural, the fetal heart rate dipped… and continued to dip, and I signed the consent form for the emergency caesarean before the epidural had even been put in. Samantha D

I had syntocinon. It gave me consistent cramping in my uterus that was a fairly convincing version of labour, but it had no effect whatsoever on the dilation of the cervix. Because this was

ultimately a 'failure to progress' induction, the contractions, though painful, felt dysfunctional. Future experiences of spontaneous, natural labour allow me to now understand that what I was feeling was a uterus being over-stimulated, but not actually achieving anything beyond wearing itself out. The obstetrician confirmed the latter when she performed my caesarean and I lost 800ml of blood – she told me this was because my uterus was 'fatigued'. A side-effect of induction was that I had, in preparation for my next birth, to do a lot of personal work to grieve the fact that I had not experienced a 'real' labour. I then also had to address my fears that my body perhaps just couldn't labour. Tessa

My synto births were harsh. The pain was evil, hence why I call it the 'devil's juice'. From the moment I was hooked up it was painful. Being on a drip and a monitor limits my movement. I like to stay upright and active during labour, but it's nearly impossible to do. It also limited my use of water as pain relief. I had one syntocinon birth without pain relief, but with all my others I opted for gas and air. There comes a point I just can't cope with the rolling pain, it's exhausting as well. Contractions are harder, faster and longer. Also no natural endorphins are released. Transition is very quick, and there is not much break before the pushing stage. There is no birth 'high' with syntocinon. In my case, it makes my brain numb. There was no love rush when I met my babies. This feeling lasts for weeks. Also they don't warn you of the dangers of syntocinon (well I wasn't): one of them is post-partum haemorrhage, which I experienced with my fourth birth. I also experienced fetal distress with my last induction, and I was lucky enough to push him out before they reviewed me for a caesarean (fetal ejection due to fear). After having a syntocinon birth, I'm left with an enormous amount of grief and feeling of failure. Lynda

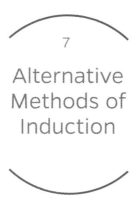

7

Alternative Methods of Induction

Induction of labour was happening long before the development of medical induction methods.[1] Today, women continue to use a variety of methods to induce labour, instead of, or in addition to, medical induction. While these approaches offer an alternative to mainstream medicine, they should not be considered 'natural'. Natural induction does not exist, because inducing a labour before it begins spontaneously is not 'natural'. All induction methods aim to initiate changes in the body to induce labour before spontaneous labour would naturally happen. Like medical methods, alternative methods of induction have side-effects and risks. Unlike medical induction, the mother and baby are not usually closely monitored with immediate access to medical support if the induction causes complications.

The effectiveness and safety of alternative induction methods is difficult to establish. Research into alternative methods is generally very limited and of poor quality. For example, many of the studies into plant-based methods have been conducted on animals, or by applying the active ingredient directly onto animal tissue in a petri dish. In these cases, the doses tested have been much higher than would normally be used by women. The studies involving humans generally only include women with a full-term pregnancy (over 37 weeks), and a 'favourable' cervix, who are therefore already close to spontaneous labour. Good quality research requires significant funding, and research funding primarily comes from industries, such as the pharmaceutical industry, with vested interests in developing a profitable product. Most alternative induction methods cannot be patented, so it is unlikely that good quality research on this topic will be funded.

Some alternative methods, such as particular aromatherapy oils, blue and black cohosh, raspberry leaf and breast stimulation, are known to stimulate uterine contractions. However, these contractions will not open the cervix unless the cervix is ripe. The use of these methods before cervical ripening can result in an extended pre-labour phase with painful, ineffective contractions, in the same way as membrane sweeping can. The result can be exhaustion, resulting in an increased need for pain relief and intervention once labour becomes established.

Another approach involves using alternative therapies to promote spontaneous labour rather than to induce labour. Stress and anxiety can inhibit oxytocin release and delay the natural start of labour. Therapies that relax the body and help to reduce stress can increase oxytocin levels. This can support the spontaneous onset of labour if it is ready to happen. Therapies such as acupuncture, Bowen therapy, massage, reflexology and particular aromatherapy oils can help women to relax and prepare for labour. This approach is distinct from attempting to induce labour before the body is ready.

This chapter provides an overview of common alternative methods of inducing labour (in alphabetical order). Instructions are not provided due to concerns about the safety of some methods, and the lack of supporting research. Alternative therapies are outside the scope of practice for midwives or doctors unless they have undertaken additional qualifications. If you choose to use alternative methods of induction, consult an appropriately qualified practitioner such as a naturopath or acupuncturist.

Alternative methods of induction

Acupuncture/Acupressure

Acupuncture is a key component of traditional Chinese medicine. It involves stimulating specific sites along the body's meridians with fine needles to encourage the normal flow of *qi* (vital energy). Induction of labour is attempted by inserting needles into sites that stimulate changes to the hormones and/or nervous system influencing the cervix and uterus. Acupressure works on the same principles, but fingers, hands or elbows are used to apply pressure to specific sites rather than needles.

A review of the available research on acupuncture found some evidence that it may help to ripen the cervix.[2] However, the overall length of labour was longer for women who received acupuncture. Another study compared acupressure with 'pretend' acupressure (pressure not applied to the correct sites) for women who were 41 weeks pregnant with their first baby.[3] The study found no difference between the groups in terms of when women went into labour, and the women who received the real acupressure were more likely to have a medical induction.

Aromatherapy

Aromatherapy oils are made by extracting aromatic essences from plants. The oils can be massaged onto the skin, added to a bath, or inhaled using a steam infuser or burner. Particular essential oils, such as jasmine and clary sage, are thought to stimulate uterine contractions. However, there is no research into the effectiveness of these oils for induction of labour. In addition, there are some concerns about these oils potentially causing excessive uterine contractions, resulting in reduced oxygen to the baby.[4]

Blue and black cohosh
Blue and black cohosh are two different plants, both native to North America, and both used for women's reproductive health. The plants can be taken as a tincture, tea, powder or capsule, and have been used both separately and combined to induce labour. There has been no research published examining either plant for induction of labour.

Blue cohosh, also known as squaw root or papoose root, is a species of the *Caulophyllum* family.[4] Blue cohosh contains components that relax muscles, and it is used to treat menstrual cramps. It also contains components that cause uterine contractions, and is used to cause abortion. Therefore, blue cohosh can both relax and contract the uterus. The side-effects associated with blue cohosh include high blood pressure and meconium-stained amniotic fluid.[5] The components of blue cohosh may also have a toxic effect on heart muscle.[4] There have been anecdotal reports of complications following the consumption of blue cohosh in pregnancy, including damage to babies' hearts.

Black cohosh, also known as black snakeroot and fairy candle, is a species of the *Ranunculacea* family.[4] It is used to treat pre-menstrual symptoms, menopausal symptoms, and to cause abortion. Black cohosh contains compounds that may reduce levels of the hormone progesterone.[6] During pregnancy high levels of progesterone relax the uterine muscle.

Before spontaneous labour begins, progesterone levels drop, contributing to the ability of the uterus to contract. The side-effects associated with black cohosh include stomach upset and low blood pressure.

Breast stimulation

Breast stimulation has been used historically, and across many cultures, to induce labour.[7] Breast stimulation is known to cause uterine contractions, most likely due to the release of oxytocin. This mechanism assists with the contraction of the uterus after birth in response to breastfeeding. In pregnancy, stimulation of both breasts at the same time has been linked to hyperstimulation of the uterus. Therefore, studies examining breast stimulation for induction have only included breast massage or nipple stimulation of one breast at a time. Studies have also involved a range of methods and frequency of breast stimulation. For example, some studies used breast pumps to stimulate the nipples, whereas most required women to manually stimulate their own breasts. Some studies required women to undertake breast stimulation for 15 minutes, three times a day; others required up to an hour a day.

A Cochrane review of all the available studies found that overall breast stimulation was effective at inducing labour, but only for women who had a full-term pregnancy and a ripe cervix.[7] Breast stimulation in combination with a ripe cervix resulted in 37% of women going into labour within 72 hours. In the group of women who did not undertake breast stimulation, only 6% were in labour within 72 hours. Breast stimulation in pregnancy also reduced the chance of haemorrhage after birth to less than 1% compared to 6% without breast stimulation. Therefore, it appears that for women who are close to spontaneous labour, breast stimulation may offer an effective method of alternative induction. However, there is insufficient research to demonstrate effectiveness or safety for women who are not full term, or who have pregnancy complications.

Castor oil

Castor oil comes from the seeds of the castor bean plant, and has been used to induce labour since as far back as ancient Egypt.[8] It can be administered by enema, but more commonly is consumed as a liquid. Castor oil is a powerful laxative; its active component, ricinoleic acid, activates prostaglandin receptors and induces contractions in the intestine and in uterine muscle.[9]

A Cochrane review of three small studies found that taking one dose (60ml) of castor oil increased women's chance of going into labour within 24 hours.[8] However, the review warns that the findings should be interpreted with caution, because the studies were of poor quality and may have been biased. In addition, all three studies also found that every woman taking castor oil experienced nausea. Other small studies have been published since the Cochrane review. The first study compared castor oil with sunflower oil for induction for post-dates pregnancies.[10] It found no differences in outcomes for women having their first baby. However, women having subsequent babies were more likely to go into labour within 24 hours if they had castor oil (60%) compared to sunflower oil (29%).

Curry

Curry and other spicy foods are sometimes believed to start labour. There is no research into the use of curry or spices to induce labour. Curry can cause digestive irritation, and emptying of the bowel, for some women. In theory, empty bowels may allow the baby's head to move deeper into the pelvis, where it can apply more pressure on the cervix. If the cervix has ripened and is ready for labour, this pressure may result in uterine contractions.

Dates

The three studies into the effect of dates on labour outcomes were carried out with very small samples, and are published in low-quality journals. The studies were also carried out in Iran and Jordan, where date consumption is a cultural practice.[11] Therefore, not being able to eat dates may have altered the outcomes for the women in the 'non-date-eating' groups. The first study included 69 women who ate six dates per day for four weeks before their estimated due date, and 45 women who ate no dates.[11] Women who had consumed dates were more likely to go into spontaneous labour (96%) compared to those who had not (79%). They were also less likely to have prostin or syntocinon during labour (28% compared to 43% in the 'no dates' group); were less likely to have their waters break before going to hospital (17% compared to 40%); and had shorter pre-labour phases (on average 8.5 hours compared to 15 hours).

The second study found that eating dates at the end of pregnancy was associated with a riper cervix on admission to hospital, and a decreased use of syntocinon in labour (20% compared with 45% in the 'no dates' group).[12,13] For women in this study who had their labour induced, eating dates increased their chance of a vaginal birth (47% compared to 28%). The third study examined whether eating dates immediately after the birth of the placenta reduced bleeding in the first three hours.[14] The study found that the average blood loss was lower for women who had eaten dates (162ml) compared to those who had not (220ml). Although these studies are of poor quality, they may support the idea that compounds in dates work on oxytocin receptors in the uterus and improve their response to syntocinon and/or create contractions. However, further high-quality research is needed to determine this.

Evening primrose oil

Evening primrose oil is commonly used to treat menstrual irregularities and pre-menstrual symptoms.[4] It has also been used to promote cervical ripening in order to induce labour, either by consuming it in liquid or capsule form, or by applying it directly to the cervix. There is only one study examining the effect of evening primrose oil on the length of pregnancy.[15] The study compared the outcomes for women who consumed evening primrose oil from 37 weeks' gestation with women who did not. Evening primrose oil did not shorten the length of pregnancy, or decrease the overall length of labour. The study also found that evening primrose oil increased the chance of prolonged rupture of membranes, the use of syntocinon to speed labour up, and vacuum delivery.

Homeopathic remedies

Homeopathy is a system of alternative medicine developed by Samuel Hahnermann in the 17–1800s.[6] It is based on the Law of Similars, that 'like cures like', and aims to correct symptoms of ill-health by using substances that produce similar symptoms in healthy people, thereby stimulating the body's own self-healing response. Homeopathic remedies are derived from herbs, minerals and other naturally occurring substances. These substances are repeatedly diluted, and the final remedies may contain very few single molecules of the original substance, or none at all. These highly diluted remedies are thought to produce results more quickly and without side-effects. The remedies are taken in tablet form or diluted in water. The most common homeopathic remedies used to induce labour are preparations of blue cohosh (*caulophyllum thalictroides*) and black cohosh (*actaea racemosa*). A Cochrane review examined the available research comparing homeopathy for induction with a placebo.[16] Only two studies were reviewed and no differences in outcomes were found between the homeopathy group and the placebo group.

Hypnosis

Hypnosis involves using a relaxation technique to create an altered state of consciousness. In this state the person is receptive to suggestions. A Cochrane review found only one study examining hypnosis for induction, and this study was of insufficient quality to be reviewed.[17]

Pineapple

Pineapple, like mango and papaya, contains bromelain, which is thought to both relax smooth muscle, and to stimulate smooth muscle to induce labour.[4] However, studies also suggest that bromelain reduces the level of prostaglandins, a hormone associated with ripening the cervix. There are currently no studies examining pineapple or bromelain for induction of labour. In addition, bromelain should be avoided when taking particular medications, for example anti-coagulants (blood thinners) and some antibiotics.

Raspberry leaf

Raspberry leaf is consumed as a tea or in a tablet. It is believed that raspberry leaf tones the uterus, encouraging labour to begin, and making contractions more effective once labour starts.[4] Raspberry leaf may not be considered a method of induction because it 'prepares' the uterus for spontaneous labour. However, the body prepares the uterus itself for labour, and does not require additional interventions to do this. Lots of changes take place in the uterus and cervix at the end of pregnancy, orchestrated by the natural hormones of pregnancy (see chapter 4).

In studies using animal uterine tissue, raspberry leaf has

been found to relax contracted uterine muscle, and contract relaxed uterine muscle.[18] Therefore, the action of the plant may depend upon the state of the muscle at the time of administration. This helps to explain why raspberry leaf is also used to relieve menstrual cramps. However, applying raspberry leaf directly onto uterine tissue is very different to delivering it via the blood system by consuming it. There is very little research into the outcomes associated with consuming raspberry leaf in pregnancy. The studies available found no evidence that raspberry leaf reduces the length of pregnancy, or speeds up labour.[18] Some women experience strong Braxton Hicks contractions after consuming raspberry leaf. Therefore, it is not recommended for women who have had a previous pre-term labour, or a previous fast labour.

Reflexology

Reflexology involves the application of pressure to specific sites on the body located on the feet, hands and outer ears to restore the flow of energy (*qi*). It is based on the idea that there are reflexes in these areas of the body that directly relate to the organs and nervous system. Therefore, stimulating these reflexes can affect other areas of the body and improve health. Some early studies found that regular reflexology increased the likelihood of spontaneous labour.[4] However, there are inadequate good-quality studies in this area to determine the effectiveness of this therapy.

Sexual intercourse

In theory there are a number of reasons why sexual intercourse may assist in initiating labour. Human semen contains high levels of prostaglandin, a substance known to assist in ripening the cervix. Oxytocin, the hormone that initiates uterine contractions, is released during sex, orgasm and nipple stimulation. In addition, sexual intercourse may stimulate the cervix. However, there is no research to support the use of sexual intercourse for induction of labour.[19]

Walking
Walking combines movement with an upright position, creating downward pressure from the baby onto the cervix. Many women find that they experience increased Braxton Hicks (non-labour) contractions when they walk during pregnancy. A survey asking women what started their labour found that 32% reported that physical activity, primarily walking, triggered their labour.[20] However, there are no good-quality studies examining physical activity for induction of labour.

I was 42 weeks pregnant the day I decided to try blue cohosh. I had been to the hospital for a wellbeing CTG [cardiotocograph], and the baby was well. But I was well aware that I would lose my place at the birth centre if I didn't have the baby in the next few days. I had negotiated a medical induction at 42+3. As is a pattern for me now, I started to go a little bit crazy just before labour, and when I got home from the hospital that day I started to google induction methods. I came across blue cohosh and read everything I could. I decided it was worth the risk, and called a naturopathic clinic to get some. They were unfamiliar with using it for induction, and didn't have much advice for me on how to use it, other than to start slow, which I did. Almost straight away I started to have light contractions, which stopped me from being able to have a sleep that afternoon. I continued on into the evening and morning, and the next night. I ended up with an emergency caesarean nearly 48 hours after I took my first dose, and for me it was the first intervention in the cascade. My next three births were uncomplicated HBACs [home birth after caesarean].

When I was compelled to 'do' something in my next pregnancies, I wrote letters to my babies, hugged my belly and was grateful I carried my children to full term, and tried to be grateful for the last few days that I was granted with a baby in my belly. Belinda

At 44 weeks my midwife suggested a massage on my sacrum with undiluted clary sage oil, which I agreed to, and within literally five minutes my waves had begun and I had my baby 2.5 hours later, healthy and perfect. Jessica

I find it funny how I never saw these alternate methods as induction. Even after my horrific experience with the first being medically induced, I was all about raspberry tea and acupuncture with my second. I still see alternate and medical induction in such different lights. Meg

I tried alternative methods. Including sex, acupuncture, walking up hills, one foot up and one foot down on a gutter, and stairs. I tried dried dates, and raspberry leaf tea. Nothing worked. I was trying to avoid medical induction. Kym

With my fourth I was determined to get it going. I had had about four weeks of heavy Braxton Hicks contractions, three weeks of night-time contractions fizzling out by morning. For three nights in a row before the birth I had hardly slept a wink because I had to breathe through irregular contractions all night. I walked and did stairs, I had taken evening primrose, I was drinking raspberry leaf tea, having acupressure and acupuncture. I also had sex. Nothing worked! In the end, the day before the birth, a friend recommended black cohosh. She was a doula, and I trusted her with this information. Even upon reading I was a bit hesitant, but was willing to try anything by this stage. Ultimately my baby literally flew out after medical induction, but I had a large postpartum haemorrhage, and I feel the cohosh may have been the trigger for that.   *Samantha D*

I strongly believe the stars aligned for my third birth, or rather the fear subsided and the oxytocin levels increased to enable my body to do what it needed to birth my baby. And I believe the reflexology treatment that I had strongly influenced everything for me. Along with the treatment she used clary sage, but also spoke through a beautiful relaxation about letting go. I needed this so much. I had three membrane sweeps, plus the amazing induction treatment from the reflexologist. I woke up on the morning of the planned induction day and my waters broke. No one went near me, and I had an amazing water birth that evening.   *Alice*

I declined all offers of stretch and sweeps and agreed for a scan at 42 weeks to make a plan if I reached that point. Earlier in my pregnancy I had thought I'd try some natural induction methods, but as the third trimester got to the pointy end, it never felt right to try any of them. In fact, I cancelled acupuncture from 38 weeks (I'd been having it since 31 weeks) because I was terrified of going into labour while driving home. It turns out I didn't need any of them, and had a physiological birth at 41 weeks.   *Helen*

With my third I tried eating dates, acupressure, nipple stimulation using an electric double breast pump, and clary sage massaged into my abdomen and lower back. Then my waters broke before labour started, so I used the double breast pump to get contractions going. I had been trying to avoid a pregnancy that went beyond 42 weeks as I was in a publicly-funded home birth programme so had restrictions on what the midwives could do. The breast pump was actually successful. After I started getting contractions that petered out after daybreak, I used the pump and started contracting within five minutes. Unfortunately, I got a migraine soon after so I stopped pumping to sleep it off. A few hours later I tried with the pump again, and got myself into good labour, birthing less than three hours later. I was trying to avoid a transfer to hospital for prolonged rupture of membranes, where I would be offered IV antibiotics and an augmentation of labour to expedite the birth. I was really happy the breast pump worked!   Anna

My induction was through acupuncture. Around the time of my due date things were very hectic in our lives as we had bought our first home, and moved house the day after I was due. I really didn't feel I had the opportunity to 'nest' and get myself into a good head space so labour could start naturally. My induction was booked for nine days overdue at my 40-week appointment, which made me feel like I was on the clock and running out of time to let my body do things itself. When I was four days overdue I booked an appointment with a friend of mine who is a chiropractor and acupuncturist. He saw me straight away as I was experiencing a lot of pain in my lower back and down my leg. He told me about his experiences of inducing other women through acupuncture, and I was keen to give it a go. The next morning at 9.30am I started having contractions, and I had my baby in the early hours of the next morning.   Hannah

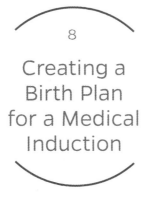

8

Creating a Birth Plan for a Medical Induction

Having your labour induced can be a positive and empowering experience. Agreeing to an induction does not mean you have signed over control of your body, or your birth. You can make the decision to have an induction, and you can make decisions about how your induction is carried out. Writing a birth plan can help you to consider your options, and communicate your choices to your care providers and support people. Although a birth plan is a blueprint and may be subject to change, writing one allows you to state your intentions for your labour experience. It is helpful for your care providers to know what your intentions and choices are so that they can help you to achieve them where possible. A birth plan can also be useful for your support people to use as a basis for advocating for you.

This chapter will help you write a birth plan specifically for induction of labour. It is hoped that the suggestions offered, and questions posed, will help you to consider your options and ultimately decide what is best for you. You might like to use the subheadings in this chapter to create a framework for your birth plan, writing statements and bullet points under each heading. It is best to keep your birth plan concise and clear, so that your care providers can quickly read and understand what you want. It is also a good idea to write your plan using clear and positive statements rather than negative statements. Focus on what you do want, rather than what you don't want. For example, 'I would like to wait for at least two hours after having my waters broken before deciding if syntocinon is needed', rather than 'I do not want syntocinon immediately after having my waters broken'. Choose wording you are comfortable with: 'want', or 'like', or 'prefer'. Don't be apologetic about having strong ideas about what you want, and remember that you are not obliged to provide reasons for your decisions. This is your body, your baby, and your birth experience. Also avoid statements such as '...unless medically indicated'. Instead, state at the beginning of your birth plan that any changes must be fully explained before you will consent to them (see below). The definition of 'medically indicated' is subjective, and your perception may be different to your care providers'. Some women create visual birth plans using graphics available free online (google 'visual birth plan graphics'). However, some graphics include options that are specific to the United States, for example, eye ointment for babies.

Ideally, your birth plan can be discussed with your care provider before your induction begins. It is also helpful to know about particular hospital guidelines (see the questions below) so that you can decide beforehand if you want to follow them. Guidelines should be publicly accessible and/or you can ask about them at an antenatal appointment. Make three copies of your birth plan: one for your support person/s; one for your hand-held maternity notes; and one for your hospital maternity notes. If you have created a visual birth plan, it can be placed on the door to your birth room. Most care providers are familiar with birth plans and will ask if you have one. If not, you or your support person will need to direct them to the birth plan in your maternity notes.

Birth plan for a medical induction of labour

1. Decision making

Start your birth plan with a clear statement about your expectations regarding roles and responsibilities in decision-making (see chapter 1).

> *Statement example:* 'I understand that it is the role of health professionals to share relevant, evidence-based information with me to assist in my decision making, and to gain consent for procedures. I also understand that my decisions, and any outcomes resulting from my decisions, are my own responsibility.'

During your induction there may be a need to reconsider and/or change your birth plan. How do you want your care providers to help you make decisions if this happens? Do you want to use the BRAIN framework – Benefits, Risks, Alternatives, Intuition, Now/Nothing (see chapter 1)? While you can consider the 'intuition' element yourself, your care providers can help to inform you about the other elements.

> *Statement example:* 'I understand that this birth plan, and my preferences, might change, and I will inform my care provider if I want to make any changes. If my care provider recommends any changes to my birth plan I would like information about:
> • the benefits and risks of the suggested change

- whether I need to make the decision immediately
- what may happen if I choose not to follow the recommendation.

Before making my decision I would like to be left alone to discuss my options with my support person/s.'

2. Ripening the cervix

After reading 'ripening the cervix' (chapter 5), consider the following questions and write down your preferences for this phase of the induction process:

Support person/s

Ripening the cervix can take many hours, and in some cases days. You may choose a different support person for this phase of the process, or the same one as you plan to have with you during labour. If you are staying in hospital overnight, will this person stay with you, or will they go home? If they go home, when would you like them to return?

Method of cervical ripening

The method of cervical ripening should have been discussed and agreed with you prior to your admission to hospital. You should also know how long there will be between the prostin administration, or balloon insertion, and the next assessment. It is worth writing this down so that your care provider can confirm your understanding, or explain any changes.

Comfort measures/pain relief

Most women experience some pain and discomfort with prostins and balloon catheters. What are your preferences for pain relief, for example, hot packs, warm shower, pain medications such as paracetamol? Sedatives are sometimes offered to help women to sleep overnight while waiting for the prostin or balloon to take effect. Would you consider taking a sedative to help you sleep? Do you prefer other methods that help you sleep, for example herbal tea, lavender essential oil, or your own pillow? You can bring these into hospital with you.

Waiting for ripening to work
What will you do after the prostin or balloon catheter has been administered? Is there a hospital guideline recommending that you stay in hospital? Will you feel safer and/or more comfortable staying in hospital or going home? If you choose to stay in hospital would you like to go outside for a walk, or to have lunch/dinner with your support person?

3. Breaking the waters
After reading 'breaking the waters' (chapter 5), consider the following questions and write down your preferences:

After artificial rupture of membranes (ARM)
After ARM do you want to start syntocinon straight away? Do you want to wait and see if you start to have contractions without syntocinon? If you want to wait, how long will you wait? What will you do while you wait? Walking can help the baby's head move down and press on the cervix, which may start contractions.

Meconium-stained amniotic fluid
It is common for meconium to be in the amniotic fluid after 41 weeks (see pages 64–66). What will you do if there is meconium in your amniotic fluid? Are there any additional interventions recommended in the hospital guidelines for meconium-stained amniotic fluid? Do you agree with the recommendations?

4. Syntocinon-induced labour

If you go into labour without syntocinon, your labour may be very similar to a spontaneous labour. However, a syntocinon-induced labour requires some additional considerations. Read chapter 6, consider the following and write down your preferences:

Environment and interactions

The environment around you influences how you feel, and how your labour progresses. You can create an environment that helps your body to release your own oxytocin to minimise the amount of syntocinon needed. Privacy, low lighting, minimal distractions and feeling safe and loved all increase oxytocin release. Consider the kind of environment and interactions that will help you to feel relaxed and safe. Write them down, and be specific, for example 'I want the birth room door closed'.

How your care providers interact with you can also influence how you feel, and therefore your labour. It can be helpful to include a statement about how you want your care providers to interact with you during labour. Do you want them to speak quietly, and only when necessary? Or do you want them to offer lots of conversation and/or reassurance? Before carrying out routine observations, such as checking your blood pressure, do you want them to ask every time? Or can they approach you to start, and if it is not OK you will indicate that by moving away? If other staff members wish to enter your birth room, do you want to be asked permission first?

Intravenous cannula (IV)

You will have an IV inserted before starting your syntocinon infusion. It is best to have your cannula inserted so that it does not inhibit the movement of your hand, or catch on things as you move around. You can request that the cannula is put into your non-dominant arm. Placing the cannula in the top of your forearm, near your wrist (where a watch is worn) allows you to move your hand easily without discomfort.

Pain management

Induced contractions are generally more painful than spontaneous contractions. Do you know about the pain relief options available, or do you need your care provider to tell you about each option in detail? Do you want your care provider to offer pain relief if they think you need it, or do you want them to wait until you ask for it? Do you want to start with no pain relief, or the least strong method, and move on to stronger methods if, and when you need them? An epidural is the only method that can completely relieve pain during labour (if it works effectively). If you know you want an epidural, do you want it set up and working before the syntocinon infusion starts?

Management of syntocinon infusion

Do you want your syntocinon turned down or off once your contraction pattern is established (see page 111)? It is very likely that your contractions will slow down or stop if you do this. However, in some cases natural oxytocin levels are high enough to continue making effective contractions. The syntocinon infusion can be increased again if your contractions reduce.

Cardiotocograph (CTG) monitoring)

Continuous CTG monitoring is recommended during an induction because of the potential effects of syntocinon (see chapter 6). If you decline CTG monitoring with syntocinon, your care provider is likely to stop administering syntocinon.

This is because it is considered unsafe to administer a medication without being able to monitor the effects of the medication on you and your baby.

However, there are options for you to consider about CTG monitoring. Find out what type of monitoring equipment is available. If the hospital has cordless waterproof CTG, you may be able to use it in the shower. If the monitor available requires you to be connected to cords, you will still be able to stand up and move around next to the monitor. You do not need to stay on the bed unless you have an epidural. If you want to use a birth ball, a mattress on the floor, or a beanbag while being monitored, write this in your birth plan. Your care provider can work around you to get a CTG reading. Consider if you want the monitor sound turned down to avoid being distracted by it. Or will you be reassured by hearing your baby's heart rate? Do you want every heart rate pattern change explained, or do you only want to know if there is a concern?

Assessing progress
It is important to know that syntocinon-induced contractions are opening the cervix. Vaginal examinations can confirm whether the rate of syntocinon is effective or not. However, you can still decline vaginal examinations if you wish. You may decide to only have a vaginal examination if the baby is not born within a particular timeframe, or if there are any concerns about progress or wellbeing. Your care provider will be able to assess the position of your baby, and whether he or she is moving downwards, by palpating your bump. On the other hand, you may want to know what your cervix is doing, and therefore want vaginal examinations. You can also use your birth plan to document any preferences about how a vaginal examination is carried out, for example, whether you want your care provider to explain what they find as they do

the examination, or to wait until they have finished and you are comfortable. You may also choose not to be told specifics (e.g. centimetres dilated), but rather be told whether you are progressing well or not.

Pushing baby out
There are differences in the pushing phase of a syntocinon-induced labour compared to a spontaneous labour. These differences can increase the chance of complications occurring (see chapter 6). However, there are some strategies you can include in your birth plan that can help to reduce the risks of syntocinon.

You can request that the syntocinon is turned down to create more space in between contractions. This will provide more recovery time for your baby between pushes. However, if your contractions become weaker it may be best to turn it back up again.

Pushing that is directed by your care provider increases the chance that your baby will become distressed, and increases your chance of perineal tearing.[1] Unfortunately, directed pushing is still a common practice. Therefore, you can include a statement in your birth plan to communicate what you would like to happen while you push. For example, 'I would like to follow my own bodily urges when I push my baby out. I would like my care provider/s to give me non-directive, reassuring support as I do this.' Or you may prefer that everyone remains silent as you push your baby out.

If you have an epidural you may wish to have it turned down so that you can feel some pushing urges. However, this is not necessary, because babies can be born without any pushing as the uterus moves the baby down with contractions. If you do want some direction to assist you to push with an epidural, waiting until the baby is low enough in your vagina to be able to see the top of his/her head before pushing reduces the risks of directed pushing.[2]

Consider birth positions that increase the size of your pelvis and reduce the pressure and stretch in your perineum, for example, kneeling on all fours or lying on your side. Avoid a semi-reclined position because it increases the chance of tearing.[3] If you have an epidural you may need some assistance to get into a good birth position. For example, it is usually possible with an epidural to kneel and lean over the back of the bed. If you are unable to kneel, a side-lying position can reduce the chance of tearing.[3]

Some care providers pull on the baby's head to deliver the baby's body as soon as the head is born. You can request that your care provider does not touch or pull on your baby during the birth. You can also state in your birth plan that you, or your support person, will be the first person to touch the baby and lift him or her up to you.

In some cases, particularly during an induction for a complication, a paediatrician will be required by hospital guidelines to attend the birth. However, the paediatrician does not need to be in the room during the birth. They can wait outside and only come in if the baby requires treatment. This helps to maintain a private birth space. You can request this in your birth plan.

5. The first hours after birth
Meeting your baby
How would you like to meet your baby? Do you want the environment to remain dimly lit and calm? Do you want to discover the sex of your baby yourself? Immediate skin-to-skin is standard practice in most hospitals. However, it can often be hurried or overlooked. You can include a statement about skin-to-skin in your birth plan, for example: 'I want my

baby to remain in undisturbed skin-to-skin contact with me until I request otherwise. I am happy to delay routine checking and weighing of my baby until later.'

Unlike oxytocin, syntocinon does not promote bonding behaviours between mother and baby (see chapter 6). However, you can increase your oxytocin, and your baby's oxytocin, by interacting with your baby. Looking at, touching, smelling and talking to your baby all promote oxytocin release. Allowing your baby to crawl to your breasts and stimulate your nipples with their hands and mouth also increases oxytocin. Skin-to-skin contact between you and your baby is not just for immediately after birth. You can hold your baby skin-to-skin as often, and for as long as you want. You may also wish to delay visitors and disturbances to allow you focused time alone with your baby.

Birthing the placenta

Active management of the placenta is required if you have had syntocinon in labour to prevent excessive bleeding (see page 119). Read page 112 and consider the following options for the birth of your placenta.

When do you want the additional bolus of syntocinon given? It is usually given immediately after the birth of the baby. However, giving it after the birth of the placenta still reduces the chance of excessive bleeding.[4] You can request to have it given after the umbilical cord has stopped pulsing so that the medication is not transferred through the placenta to your baby.

When do you want your baby's cord to be clamped? The transfer of baby's blood from the placenta usually takes around three minutes (see pages 90–91). You can request that the cord is only cut after it has stopped pulsing and is completely white (empty). Or, you could ask to wait until after the placenta is born (it is possible to do active management with the cord still attached to the baby). Or, you may wish to write a statement that ensures your care providers wait for your agreement before clamping and cutting the cord, then decide at the time. For example: 'Even if resuscitation is required, wait until I have given explicit verbal consent before cutting my baby's umbilical cord'.

Many care providers immediately clamp and cut the cord of a baby who requires resuscitation. However, it is more effective to resuscitate a baby who is still attached to their placenta and therefore receiving oxygen, and their full blood volume.[5] Find out what the common practice is at your hospital. You may need to write in your birth plan that any resuscitation should take place with the cord intact. Resuscitation equipment can be brought to your baby rather than taking your baby away.

If baby goes to special care nursery

If your baby goes to special care nursery, for whatever reason, it can be very helpful to have a written plan about what you would like to happen. Consider the following.

Who will go with your baby initially until you are able to visit? Do you consent to any medications being given to your baby, or do you want staff to discuss this with you first? How are you planning to feed your baby? Do you have some expressed breastmilk ready, just in case? Would you like help to express some breastmilk for your baby as soon as possible after birth? If you do not want your baby to have formula, include a statement such as: 'Only give my baby formula after explaining the reason it is recommended, and gaining my consent.'

6. Caesarean

A caesarean is a common outcome of induction, particularly for women having their first baby. Any caesarean carried out during labour without prior planning is classified as an 'emergency' caesarean. However, a very sudden and rushed caesarean is rare. Usually, there is some prior warning that a caesarean is looking likely, and time to prepare. It can be helpful to find out about caesarean birth and write a plan for this scenario. For example, including details about who you want with you in theatre as your support person, and how you want your care providers to interact with you. Have you brought specific music you would like played in theatre? Do you want theatre staff to avoid having personal conversations that are unrelated to the birth? Do you want to watch your baby emerge? Do you want to discover the sex for yourself? Do you want your baby brought directly to you? Theatre is often cold, but you can have your baby put skin-to-skin immediately after birth to keep them warm.

A baby born by caesarean misses out on being colonised by vaginal microbiota, which alters their microbiome. Some women take a vaginal swab with a clean cloth before surgery to wipe over their baby after birth. Care providers are becoming increasingly familiar with the process of 'vaginal seeding' for caesarean babies. It may be worth discussing this with your care provider before labour.

Messages from mothers who have experienced induction

Dear mother: sometimes induction is the best choice for you and your baby, you don't need to feel bad about it. Ask your care provider to start with the least invasive procedures and learn how help your body and your baby in the process. Ask to be up, change position, sing and do whatever you want. Even in an induction, you can guide the process and make it your own. Inform yourself and your partner about all the steps of the process. You can do this! A doula may help you with everything, and remind you during the induction what you can do to make it more effective. Remember, your body, your baby, your choice.   *Mariana*

It's ok to say no! Remember this is your birth and your experience! Look at all options. If you're unsure of something, ask! I was able to guide the induction process with the support of my caregivers. I requested to wait after an ARM prior to syntocinon, and although I still required syntocinon, I am grateful that I was able to give my body some time. My birth was still beautiful; we had delayed cord clamping and hours of skin-to-skin. It truly was a wonderful experience.   *Tracey*

I was so glad that I told my partner to ask the hospital staff to leave any time a decision had to be made on the day. It meant we could take in the facts and options presented, and make a decision together about consent without the added pressure of the hospital staff. Don't accept generalised statements like 'it's hospital protocol'. Find out why.   *Meg*

Don't let anyone talk you out of a birth plan. Yes some are unrealistic, but if you don't write your wishes down you can't guarantee that all the staff will know what you want. It's also a good discussion point to see if your expectations will be able to fit with the induction methods used.   *Linda*

Access a doula, or the best birth support that you can. Look deep into the eyes of each of your care providers and clearly state you are going to birth as naturally as possible and ask them if they can truly support you with that. If it's clear (or subtle) that they can't, then you can ask for a care provider who can. Prepare yourself mentally and spiritually, meditate with your baby, connect with the divine, whatever that means to you. Get into as clear, determined, strong and happy a state as you can, let go of all fear as much as you can, and embrace The Great Yes. Doing these things helped me to have a life-changing, beautiful induced birth and I wish you great blessings for your birth.　　*Lana*

Use the BRAIN acronym [see chapter 1]. Ask about the benefits, risks, alternatives, your instincts and what if you do nothing/ wait to help you make an informed decision and be able to trust that this is the right decision for the birth of your baby. With my first labour, I wish I hadn't stayed on the bed and then birthed on my back. I still had a beautiful straightforward birth, but my body would have birthed much easier if I had been on all fours or more mobile like I was in my second induction – I was so glad I had the ARM and then waited a couple of hours before syntocinon because I didn't need it.　　*Alice*

My first birth ended up in an emergency caesarean after syntocinon. I didn't make a birth plan. I wasn't even told it was a good idea to do one just in case. I had birth trauma from the birth. I went on to have three vaginal births after this. For my fifth birth, I planned on a natural birth but instinctively I knew it would be a caesarean. This time I clearly told the midwives, doctors and anaesthesist about my previous trauma, and what I wanted and did not want verbally. Everything was followed and I had an emotionally positive experience. I would highly recommend ALL women think about the possibility of 'what if', and clearly express their wishes to birthing partners, and have it on paper in the event it goes that way. It's not being negative. It is being prepared.　　*Samantha D*

I wrote a one-page birth plan specifically in case I had a caesarean. I also included wishes for if babe was in the nursery. I wrote that I consented to having my breastmilk expressed by a midwife if I was unconscious, and included options for donor milk if that was required.　　*Anna*

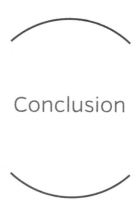

Conclusion

Induction of labour is here to stay, and in many cases it is a useful intervention that improves outcomes for women and their babies. However, it is important that individual women's needs are prioritised over health professionals' routine preferences and recommendations. Choosing to be induced, or not, is ultimately the woman's decision and no one else's. The right to choose is protected by law, and requires health professionals to provide adequate information to assist women's decision-making. Health professionals are also required to respect and support a woman's decision, regardless of whether it aligns with recommendations.

This book explored induction, from making a decision about induction, through to creating a birth plan for an induced labour. It discussed what research and guidelines say about induction, and more importantly shared what women themselves say about their experiences. Choosing whether to have your labour induced is a complex decision that should be made free of judgment or pressure from others. This book aims to help women to make their own empowered decisions about induction. For those who choose induction, the book offers honest information about what the process involves. Knowing what to expect can help with preparation, and in creating a plan to inform how your induction is carried out.

Every birth is unique and results not only in the birth of a baby, but of a mother too. If we want mothers to trust in their ability to nurture their babies and know what is best for them, we must support women to trust in their ability to make decisions about birth. It is my wish that every woman, regardless of how she gives birth, steps into motherhood feeling strong and empowered, knowing that she is the expert when it comes to her body and her baby.

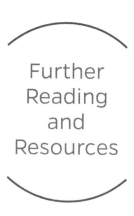

Further Reading and Resources

Association for Improvements in the Maternity Services (AIMS) *www.aims.org.uk*

Birthrights *www.birthrights.org.uk*

Gestational Diabetes UK *www.gestationaldiabetes.co.uk*

ICP Support *www.icpsupport.org*

MidwifeThinking *midwifethinking.com*

National Childbirth Trust (NCT) *www.nct.org.uk*

National Institute for Health and Care Excellence (NICE) *www.nice.org.uk*

Positive Birth Movement *www.positivebirthmovement.org*

Preeclampsia Foundation *www.preeclampsia.org*

Stillbirth and Neonatal Death Charity (SANDS) *www.sands. org.uk*

The Birth Trauma Association *www.birthtraumaassociation. org.uk*

The Cochrane Collaboration *www.cochrane.org*

Twins & Multiple Birth Association (TAMBA) *www.tamba. org.uk/pregnancy*

Acknowledgements

Firstly I would like to thank all of the women who generously contributed their personal experiences to this book. Their honest sharing has been invaluable in making this book about far more than research and guidelines.

I would also like to thank my reviewers Sarah Cornfoot, Jessie Johnson-Cash and Kendall George. I am especially thankful to my husband Duncan Reed, who not only read my drafts, but also provided tea, cake and encouragement throughout.

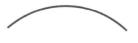

References

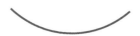

Introduction

1. 'WHO recommendations for induction of labour', World Health Organization (2011), available at: http://www.who.int/reproductivehealth/publications/maternal_perinatal_health/9789241501156/en/ [accessed 16 January 2018].

Chapter 1

1. 'Inducing labour: clinical guideline', NICE (2014), available at: https://www.nice.org.uk/guidance/cg70 [accessed 7 December 2017].

2. Bechara, A., Damasio, H., Damasio, A.R., 'Emotion, decision making and the orbitofrontal cortex', *Cerebral Cortex* (2000), 10(3), pp. 295-307.

3. 'Caesarean section: consent advice no. 7', Royal College of Obstetricians and Gynaecologists (2009), available at: https://www.rcog.org.uk/en/guidelines-research-services/guidelines/consent-advice-7/ [accessed 7 December 2017].

4. 'Using the BRAIN worksheet for informed decision making', Centre for Collaboration, Motivation & Innovation (2016), available at: https://centrecmi.ca/2017/08/15/using-the-brain-worksheet-for-informed-decision-making/ [accessed 7 December 2017].

Chapter 2

1. 'Hypertension in pregnancy: diagnosis and management: clinical guideline', NICE (2010), available at: https://www.nice.org.uk/guidance/cg107 [accessed 13 December 2017].

2. Koopmans, C.M., et al, 'Induction of labour versus expectant monitoring for gestational hypertension or mild pre-eclampsia after 36 weeks (HYPITAT): a multicenter, open-label randomised controlled trial', *The Lancet* (2009), 374(3), pp. 979-988.

3. 'Diabetes in pregnancy: management from preconception to the postnatal period: NICE guideline', NICE (2015), available at: https://www.nice.org.uk/guidance/cg63 [accessed 13 December 2017].

4. Gregory, R., Todd, D., 'Endocrine disorders', In: Robson, S.E., Waugh, J. (eds) *Medical disorders in pregnancy: a manual for midwives* (West Sussex: John Wiley & Sons Ltd, 2013).

5. Mischke, M., Plösch, T., 'More than just a gut instinct – the potential interplay between a baby's nutrition, its gut microbiome, and the epigenome', *American Journal of Physiology-Regulatory, Integrative and Comparative Physiology* (2013), 304, pp. R1065-R1069.

6. Forester, D.A, et al, 'Safety and efficacy of antenatal milk expressing for women with diabetes in pregnancy: a protocol for a randomised controlled trial', *BMJ Open* (2014) 4:e006571. doi:10.1136/bmjopen-2014- 006571.

7. Rosenstein, M.G., et al, 'The risk of stillbirth and infant death stratified by gestational age in women with gestational diabetes', *American Journal of Obstetrics and Gynecology* (2012), 206(4), pp. 309.e1-309.e7.

8. Biesty, L.M., et al, 'Planned birth at or near term for improving health outcomes for pregnant women with gestational diabetes and their infant', *Cochrane Database of Systematic Reviews* (2018), Issue 1. Art. No.: CD004735. DOI: 10.1002/14651858.CD004735.pub4.

9. 'WHO recommendations for induction of labour', World Health Organization (2011), available at: http://www.who.int/reproductivehealth/publications/maternal_perinatal_health/9789241501156/en/ [accessed 13 December 2017].

10. 'Gestational diabetes mellitus', Queensland Clinical Guidelines (2015), available at: https://www.health.qld.gov.au/__data/assets/pdf_file/0023/140099/g-gdm.pdf [accessed 13 December 2017].

11. Murphy, H.R. et al, 'Improved outcomes in women with type 1

and type 2 diabetes but substantial clinic-to-clinic variations: a prospective nationwide study' *Diabetologia* (2017), 60, pp. 1668-1677.

12. 'About ICP', ICP Support Organisation, available at: http://www.icpsupport.org [accessed 13 December 2017].

13. 'Obstetric cholestasis: green-top guideline no. 43', RCOG (2011), available at: https://www.rcog.org.uk/en/guidelines-research-services/guidelines/gtg43/ [accessed 13 December 2013].

14. Wikström Shemer, E., Marschall, H.U., Ludvigsson, J.F., Stephansson, O., 'Intrahepatic cholestasis of pregnancy and associated adverse pregnancy and fetal outcomes: a 12 year population-based cohort study', *BJOG* (2013), DOI: 10.1111/1471-0528.12174.

15. Geenes, V., et al, 'Association of severe intrahepatic cholestasis of pregnancy with adverse pregnancy outcomes: a prospective population-based case-control study', *Hepatology* (2014), 59(4), pp.1482-1491.

16. Puljic, A., et al, 'The risk of infant and fetal death by each additional week of expectant management in intrahepatic cholestasis of pregnancy by gestational age', *American Journal of Obstetrics and Gynecology* (2015), 212, pp. 667.e5.

17. Williamson, C., et al, 'Bile acid signaling in fetus tissues: implications for intrahepatic cholestasis of pregnancy', *Digestive Diseases* (2011), 29(1), pp. 58-61.

18. Gurung, V., et al, 'Interventions for treating cholestasis in pregnancy', *Cochrane Database of Systematic Reviews* (2013), Issue 6. Art. No.: CD000493. DOI: 10.1002/14651858.CD000493.pub2.

19. Glantz, A., Marschall, H-U., Mattsson, L-A., 'Intrahepatic cholestasis of pregnancy: relationships between bile acid levels and fetal complication rates', *Hepatology* (2004), 40(2), pp. 467-474.

20. Gardosi, J., Madurasinghe, V., Williams, M., Malik, A., Francis, A., 'Maternal and fetal risk factors for stillbirth: population based study', *BMJ* (2013), doi: 10.1136/bmj.f108.

21. Francis, A., Tonks, A., Gardosi, J., 'Accuracy of ultrasound estimation of fetal weight at term', *Arch Dis Child Fetal Neonatal Ed* (2011), 91, doi: 10.1136/adc.2011.300161.24

22. Berkley, E., Chauhan, S.P., Abuhamad, A., 'Doppler assessment of the fetus with intrauterine growth restriction', *American Journal of Obstetrics and Gynecology* (2012), 206(4), pp. 300-308.

23. 'The investigation and management of the small-for-gestational-

age fetus: green-top guideline no. 31', RCOG (2014), available at: https://www.rcog.org.uk/en/guidelines-research-services/guidelines/gtg31/ [accessed 13 December 2013].

24. 'Inducing labour: clinical guideline', NICE (2014), available at: https://www.nice.org.uk/guidance/cg70 [accessed 7 December 2017]

25. 'Reduced fetal movements: green-top guideline no. 57', RCOG (2011), available at: https://www.rcog.org.uk/en/guidelines-research-services/guidelines/gtg57/ [accessed 13 December 2013].

26. PSANZ stillbirth and neonatal death alliance, available at: https://sanda.psanz.com.au [accessed 13 December 2013].

27. Pasquier, J-C., Bujold, E., 'A systematic review of intentional delivery in women with preterm prelabor rupture of membranes', *The Journal of Maternal-Fetal & Neonatal Medicine* (2007), 20(7), pp. 567-568.

28. Kenyon, S., Boulvain, M., Neilson, J.P., 'Antibiotics for preterm rupture of membranes', *Cochrane Database of Systematic Reviews* (2013), Issue 12. Art. No.: CD001058. DOI: 10.1002/14651858.CD001058.pub3.

29. Bond, D.M., et al, 'Planned early birth versus expectant management for women with preterm prelabour rupture of membranes prior to 37 weeks' gestation for improving pregnancy outcome', *Cochrane Database of Systematic Reviews* (2017), Issue 3. Art. No.: CD004735. DOI: 10.1002/14651858.CD004735.pub4.

30. Lamont, K., Scott, N.W., Jones, G.T., Bhattacharya, S., 'Risk of recurrent stillbirth: systematic review and meta-analysis', *BMJ* (2015), doi: 10.1136/bmj.h3080

Chapter 3

1. 'Childhood mortality in England and Wales: 2015', ONS (2017), available at: bit.ly/2fA7Hi3 [accessed 2 January 2018]

2. Redmond. M., *When the drummers were women: a spiritual history of rhythm* (New York: Three Rivers Press, 1997).

3. Donnison, J., *Midwives and medical men: a history of the struggle for the control of childbirth* (London: Historical Publications, 1988).

4. Dekker, R.L., 'Labour induction for later-term or post-term pregnancy', *Women and Birth* (2016), 29(4), pp. 394-398.

5. Khambalia, A.Z., et al, 'Predicting date of birth and examining the best time to date a pregnancy', *International Journal of Gynecology and Obstetrics* (2013), 123, pp. 105-109.

6. Smith, G.S.S., 'Use of time to event analysis to estimate the normal duration of human pregnancy', *Human Reproduction* (2001), 16(7), pp. 1497-1500.

7. Hunter, L.A., 'Issues in pregnancy dating: revisiting the evidence', *Journal of Midwifery & Women's Health* (2009), 54(3), pp. 184-190.

8. Juik, A.M., Baird, D.D., Weinberg, C.R., McConnaughey, D.R., Wilcox, A.J., 'Length of human pregnancy and contributors to its natural variation', *Human Reproduction* (2013), DOI:10.1093/humrep/det297.

9. McAlpine, J.M., Scott, R., Scuffham, P.A., Perkins, A.V., Vanderlelie, J.J., 'The association between third trimester multivitamin/mineral supplements and gestational length in uncomplicated pregnancies', *Women and Birth* (2016), 29, pp.41-46.

10. Kortekaas, J.C., et al 'Recurrence rate and outcome of post-term pregnancy, a national cohort study', *European Journal of Obstetrics and Gynecology and Reproductive Biology* (2015), 193, pp. 70-74.

11. Rosenstein, M.G, et al, 'risk of stillbirth and infant death stratified by gestational age', *Obstet Gynecol* (2012), 120(1), pp.76-82.

12. Gülmezoglu, A.M., Crowther, C.A., Middleton, P., Heatley, E., 'Induction of labour for improving birth outcomes for women at or beyond term'. *Cochrane Database of Systematic Reviews* (2012), Issue 6. Art. No.: CD004945. DOI: 10.1002/14651858.CD004945.pub3.

13. Fox, H, 'Aging of the placenta', Arch Dis Child (1997), 77, pp.F171-F175.

14. Maiti, K., et al, 'Evidence that fetal death is associated with placental aging', *American Journal of Obstetrics & Gynecology* (2017) 217(4), pp. 441.e1-441.e14.

15. Madruzzato, G., et al, 'Guidelines for the management of postterm pregnancy', *Journal of Perinatal Medicine* (2010), pp. 111-119.

16. Unsworth, J., Vause, S., 'Meconium in labour', *Obstetrics, Gynaecology and Reproductive Medicine* (2010), 20(10), pp. 289-294.

17. Powell, S., 'Holy meconium: a potted history', *Essentially MIDIRS* (2013), 4(9), pp. 18-24.

18. Mullins, E., Lees, C., Brocklehurst, P., 'Is electronic fetal monitoring useful for all women in labour?' *BMJ* (2017), doi: 10.1136/bmj.j5423

19. Alfirevic, Z., Devane, D., Gyte, G.M.L., 'Continuous cardiotocography (CTG) as a form of electronic fetal monitoring

(EFM) for fetal assessment during labour', *Cochrane Database of Systematic Reviews* (2013), Issue 5. Art. No.: CD006066. DOI: 10.1002/14651858.CD006066.pub2.

20. 'Intrapartum care for healthy women and babies', NICE, available at: https://www.nice.org.uk/guidance/cg190 [accessed 3 January 2018].

21. 'Birth by parents' characteristics in England and Wales: 2016', ONS (2017), available at: https://www.ons.gov.uk/peoplepopulationandcommunity/birthsdeathsandmarriages/livebirths/bulletins/birthsbyparentscharacteristicsinenglandandwales/2016 [accessed 3 January 2018]

22. Page, J.M., et al, 'The risk of stillbirth and infant death by each additional week of expectant management stratified by maternal age', *American Journal of Obstetrics and Gynecology* (2013) 209(4), pp. 375.e1–375.e7.

23. 'Induction of labour at term in older mothers: scientific impact paper no. 34', RCOG (2013), available at: https://www.rcog.org.uk/en/guidelines-research-services/guidelines/sip34/

24. Knight, H.E., et al, 'Perinatal mortality associated with induction of labour versus expectant management in nulliparous women aged 35 years or over: An English national cohort study', *PLOS Medicine* (2017),14(11): e1002425.

25. 'Cesarean section rates in OECD countries in 2015 (per 100 live births)', The Statistical Portal, available at: https://www.statista.com/statistics/283123/cesarean-sections-in-oecd-countries/ [accessed 3 January 2018].

26. 'Birth after previous caesarean birth: green-top guidelines no.45', RCOG (2015), available at: https://www.rcog.org.uk/en/guidelines-research-services/guidelines/gtg45/ [accessed 3 January 2018].

27. Landon, M.B., et al, 'Risk of uterine rupture with a trial of labor in women with multiple and single prior cesarean delivery', *Obstetrics & Gynecology* (2006), 108(1), pp. 12-20.

28. Caesarean section: consent advice no.7', RCOG (2009), available at: https://www.rcog.org.uk/en/guidelines-research-services/guidelines/consent-advice-7/ [accessed 3 January 2018].

29. Hansen, A.K., Wisborg, K., Uldbjerg, N., Brink, T., 'Risk of respiratory morbidity in term infants delivered by elective caesarean section: cohort study', *BMJ* (2007), doi:10.1136/bmj.39405.539282.BE.

30. Wakeford, A., Harman, T., *The microbiome effect: how your baby's birth affects their future health* (London: Pinter & Martin Ltd, 2016).

31. Dahlen, H.G., Downe, S., Wright, M.L., Kennedy, H.P., Taylor, J.Y., 'Childbirth and consequent atopic disease: emerging evidence on epigenetic effects based on the hygiene and EPIIC hypotheses', *BMC Pregnancy and Childbirth* (2016), 16:4, DOI 10.1186/s12884-015-0768-9

32. 'Inducing labour: clinical guideline', NICE (2014), available at: https://www.nice.org.uk/guidance/cg70 [accessed 3 January 2018]

33. 'Birth characteristics in England and Wales: 2016', ONS (2017), available at: https://www.ons.gov.uk/peoplepopulationandcommunity/birthsdeathsandmarriages/livebirths/bulletins/birthcharacteristicsinenglandandwales/2016#percentage-of-babies-with-low-birthweight-remains-unchanged-since-2011 [accessed 3 January 2018]

34. Chauhan, S.P., et al, 'Suspicion and treatment of the macrosomic fetus: a review', *American Journal of Obstetrics & Gynecology* (2005), 193(2), pp. 332-346.

35. Rossi, A.C., Mullin, P., Prefumo, F., 'Prevention, management, and outcomes of macrosomia: a systematic review of literature and meta-analysis', *Obstetrics Gynecology Survey* (2013), 68(10), pp. 702-709.

36. Cheng, E.R., Declercq, E.R., Belanoff, C., Stotland, N.E., Iverson, R.E., 'Labor and delivery experiences of mothers with suspected large babies', *Maternal and Child Health Journal* (2015), DOI 10.1007/s10995-015-1776-0.

37. Moraitis, A.A., Wood, A.M., Fleming, M., Smith, G.C., 'Birth weight percentile and the risk of term perinatal death', *Obstetrics & Gynecology* (2014), 124(2 Pt 1), pp. 274-283.

38. Wiessmann-Brenner, A., et al, 'Maternal and neonatal outcomes of macrosomic pregnancies', *Medical Science Monitor* (2012), 18(9), pp. PH77-81.

39. Linder, N., et al, 'Macrosomic newborns of non-diabetic mothers: anthropometric measurements and neonatal complications', *BMJ* (2014), 99, F352-F358.

40. Politi, S., D'Emidio, L., Cignini, P., Giorlandino, M., Giorlandino, C., 'Shoulder dystocia: an evidence-based approach', *Journal of Prenatal Medicine* (2010), 4(3), pp.35-42.

41. Sadeh-Mestechkin, D., Walfisch, A., Shachar, R., Shoham-Vardi, H., Hallak, M., 'Suspected macrosomia? Better not tell', *Archives of*

Gynecology and Obstetrics (2008), 278(3), pp.225-230.

42. Blackwell, S. C., Refuerzo, J., Chadha, R., Carreno, C.A., 'Overestimation of fetal weight by ultrasound: does it influence the likelihood of cesarean delivery for labor arrest?' *American Journal of Obstetrics & Gynecology* (2009), 200(3), pp. 340 e341-343.

43. Peleg, D., Warsof, S., Wolf, M.F., Perlitz, Y., Shachar, I.B., 'Counseling for fetal macrosomia: an estimated fetal weight of 4,000g is excessively low', *American Journal of Perinatology* (2015), 32(1), pp. 71-74.

44. Boulvain, M., Irion, O., Dowswell, T., Thornton, J.G., 'Induction of labour at or near term for suspected fetal macrosomia',.*Cochrane Database of Systematic Reviews* (2016), Issue 5. Art. No.: CD000938. DOI: 10.1002/14651858.CD000938.pub2.

45. 'WHO recommendations for induction of labour', WHO (2011), available at: http://www.who.int/reproductivehealth/publications/ maternal_perinatal_health/9789241501156/en/ [accessed 3 January 2018].

46. 'Multiple pregnancy: antenatal care for twin and triplet pregnancies', NICE (2011), available at: https://www.nice.org.uk/ guidance/cg129 [accessed 3 January 2018].

47. Page, J.M., Pilliod, R.A., Snowden, J.M., Caughey, A.B., 'The risk of stillbirth and infant death by each additional week of expectant management in twin pregnancies', *American Journal of Obstetrics & Gynecology* (2015), 212(5), pp. 620e1-630e7.

48. Dodd, J., Deussen, A., Grivell, R., Crowther, C., 'Elective birth at 37 weeks' gestation for women with an uncomplicated twin pregnancy', *Cochrane Database of Systematic Reviews* (2014), Issue 2. Art. No.: CD003582. DOI:10.1002/14651858.CD003582.pub2.

49. Middleton, P., Shepherd, E., Flenady, V., McBain, R.D., Crowther, C.A., 'Planned early birth versus expectant management (waiting) for prelabour rupture of membranes at term (37 weeks or more)', *Cochrane Database of Systematic Reviews* (2017), Issue 1. Art. No.: CD005302. DOI: 10.1002/14651858.CD005302.pub3.

50. Flenady, V., King, J.F., 'Antibiotics for prelabour rupture of membranes at or near term', *Cochrane Database of Systematic Reviews* (2002), Issue 3. Art. No.: CD001807. DOI: 10.1002/14651858.CD001807.

51. Dahlen, H., Downe, S., Duff, M., Gill, G., 'Vaginal examination during normal labor: routine examination or routine intervention', *International Journal of Childbirth* (2013), 3(3), pp. 142-152.

Chapter 4

1. Sakala, C., Romano, A.M., Buckley, S.J., 'Hormonal physiology of childbearing, an essential framework for maternal-newborn nursing', *JOGNN* (2016), 45(2), pp. 265-275.

2. Uvnäs Moberg, K., *The Oxytocin Factor* (London: Pinter & Martin Ltd, 2011).

3. Mendelson, C.R., 'Minireview: fetal-maternal hormonal signaling in pregnancy and labor', *Molecular Endocrinology* (2009), 23(7), pp. 947-954.

4. Dahlen, H.G., et al, 'The EPIIC hypothesis: intrapartum effects on the neonatal epigenome and consequent health outcomes', *Medical Hypotheses* (2013), 80(5), pp. 656–662.

5. Odent, M., 'The fetus ejection reflex', *Birth* (1987), 14(2), pp. 104-105.

6. Reed, R., 'Supporting women's instinctive pushing behaviour during birth', *The Practising Midwife* (2015), 18(6), pp. 13-15.

7. Dixon, L., Skinner, J., Foureur, M., 'The emotional and hormonal pathways of labour and birth: integrating mind, body and behaviour', *New Zealand College of Midwives* (2013), 48, pp. 15-23.

8. Reed, R., Barnes M., Rowe, J., 'Women's experience of birth: childbirth as a rite of passage', *International Journal of Childbirth* (2016), 6(1), pp. 46-56.

Chapter 5

1. Kolkman, D., et al, 'The Bishop score as a predictor of labor induction success: a systematic review', *American Journal of Perinatology* (2013), 30(8), pp. 625–630.

2. Boulvain, M., Stan, C., 'Membrane sweeping for induction of labour', *Cochrane Database of Systematic Reviews* (2005), Issue 1. Art. No.: CD000451. DOI: 10.1002/14651858.CD000451.pub2.

3. Hill, M.J., et al, 'The effect of membrane sweeping on prelabor rupture of membranes', *Obstetrics and Gynecology* (2008), 111(6), pp. 1313–1319.

4. Alfirevic, Z., et al, 'Which method is best for the induction of labour? A systematic review, network meta-analysis and cost-effectiveness analysis', *Health Technology Assessment* (2016), 20(65).

5. Jozwiak, M., et al, 'Mechanical methods for induction of labour', *Cochrane Database of Systematic Reviews* (2012), Issue 3. Art. No.: CD001233. DOI: 10.1002/14651858.CD001233.pub2.

6. Smyth R.M.D., Alldred S.K., Markham C., 'Amniotomy

for shortening spontaneous labour', *Cochrane Database of Systematic Reviews* (2013), Issue 1. Art. No.: CD006167. DOI: 10.1002/14651858.CD006167.pub3.

7.   Macones, G.A., Cahill, A., Stamilio, D.M., Odibo, A.O., 'The efficacy of early amniotomy in nulliparous labor induction: a randomized controlled trial', *American Journal of Obstetrics and Gynecology* (2012), 207(5), pp. 403.e1–403.e5.

8.   Kramer, M.S., Rouleau, J., Baskett, T.F., Joseph, K.S., 'Amniotic-fluid embolism and medical induction of labour: a retrospective, population-based cohort study', *The Lancet* (2006), 368(9545), pp. 1444–1448.

9.   Fok, W., Clapp, J., Stepanchak, W., 'Fetal hemodynamic changes after amniotomy', *Acta Obstetrica et Gynecologica Scandinavia* (2005), 84, pp.166-169.

Chapter 6

1.   Odent, M.R., 'Synthetic oxytocin and breastfeeding: Reasons for testing a hypothesis', *Medical Hypotheses* (2013), 81(5), pp. 889–891.

2.   Diven, L.C., et al, 'Oxytocin discontinuation during active labor in women who undergo labor induction', *American Journal of Obstetrics and Gynecology* (2012), 207(6), pp. 471.e1-471.e8.

3.   Selo-Ojeme, D., et al, 'Is induced labour in the nullipara associated with more maternal and perinatal morbidity?', *Archives of Gynecology and Obstetrics* (2010), 284(2), pp. 337–341.

4.   Downe, S., Gyte, G.M., Dahlen, H., Singata, M., 'Routine vaginal examinations for assessing progress of labour to improve outcomes for women and babies', *Cochrane Database of Systematic Reviews* (2013), Issue 7. Art. No.: CD010088. DOI: 10.1002/14651858. CD010088.pub2.

5.   Senturk, M.B., Cakmak, Y., Gündoğdu, M., Polat, M., Atac, H., 'Does performing cesarean section after onset of labor has positive effect on neonatal respiratory disorders?, *The Journal of Maternal-Fetal and Neonatal Medicine* (2015), DOI: 10.3109/14767058.2015.1087499.

6.   Davey, M-A., King, J., 'Caesarean section following induction of labour in uncomplicated first births – a population-based cross-sectional analysis of 42,950 births', *BMC Pregnancy and Childbirth* (2016), 16(92), DOI 10.1186/s12884-016-0869-0.

7.   Rouse, D.J., Owen, J., Savage, K.G., Hauth, J.C., 'Active phase labor arrest: revisiting the 2-hour minimum', *Obstetrics and Gynecology* (2001), 98(4), pp. 550-554.

8. Landy, H.J., et al, 'Characteristics associated with severe perineal and cervical lacerations during vaginal delivery', *Obstetrics and Gynecology* (2011), 117(3), pp. 627–635.

9. Elkamil, A.I., et al, 'Induction of labor and cerebral palsy: a population-based study in Norway', *Acta Obstet Gynecol Scand* (2011), 90(1), pp. 83–91.

10. Phaneuf, S & al, E 2000, 'Loss of myometrial oxytocin receptors during oxytocin-induced and oxytocin-augmented labour', *Journal of Reproduction and Fertility* (2000), 120, pp. 91-97.

11. Bell, A.F., Erickson, E.N., Carter, C.S. 'Beyond labor: the role of natural and synthetic oxytocin in the transition to motherhood', *Journal of Midwifery and Women's Health* (2014), 59(1), pp. 35–42.

12. Kroll-Desrosiers, A.R., et al, 'Association of peripartum synthetic oxytocin administration and depressive and anxiety disorders within the first postpartum year', *Depress Anxiety* (2017), 34, pp. 137-146.

13. Dahlen, H.G., et al, 'The EPIIC hypothesis: intrapartum effects on the neonatal epigenome and consequent health outcomes', *Medical Hypotheses* (2013), 80(5), pp. 656–662.

14. Gregory, S.G., Anthopolos, R., Osgood, C.E., Grotegut, C.A., Miranda, M.L., 'Association of autism with induced or augmented childbirth in North Carolina birth record (1990-1998) and Education Research (1997-2007) databases', *JAMA Pediatrics* (2013), 167(10), p. 959.

15. Kurth, L., Haussmann, R., 'Perinatal pitocin as an early ADHD biomarker: neurodevelopmental risk', *Journal of Attention Disorders* (2011), 15(5), pp. 423-431.

Chapter 7

1. Benrubi, G.I., 'Labor induction: historic perspectives', *Clinical Obstetrics Gynecology* (2000), 43(3), pp. 429-432.

2. Mozurkewich, E., et al, 'Methods of induction of labour: a systematic review', *BMC Pregnancy and Childbirth* (2011), 11(84), http://www.biomedcentral.com/1471-2393/11/84.

3. Gregson, S., Tiran, D., Absalom, J., Older, L., Bassett, P., 'Acupressure for inducing labour for nulliparous women with post-dates pregnancy', *Complementary Therapies in Clinical Practice* (2015), 21(4), pp. 257–261.

4. Evans, M., 'Postdates pregnancy and complementary therapies', *Complementary Therapies in Clinical Practice* (2009), 15(4), pp.

220–224.

5. Steinberg, D., Beal, M.W., 'Homeopathy and women's health care', *JOGNN* (2003), 32(2), pp. 207-214.

6. Kistin, S.J., Newman, A.D., 'Induction of labor with homeopathy: a case report', *Journal of Midwifery & Women's Health* (2007), 52(3), pp. 303-307.

7. Kavanagh, J. 'Breast stimulation for cervical ripening and induction of labour (review)', *The Cochrane Collaboration*, 2010.

8. Kelly, A.J., Kavanagh, J., Thomas, J. 'Castor oil, bath and/or enema for cervical priming and induction of labour' *Cochrane Database of Systematic Reviews* (2013), Issue 7. Art. No.: CD003099. DOI: 10.1002/14651858.CD003099.pub2.

9. Tunaru, S., Althoff, T.F., Nusing, R.M., Diener, M., Offermanns, S., 'Castor oil induces laxation and uterus contraction via ricinoleic acid activating prostaglandin EP_3 receptors', *Proceedings of the National Academy of Sciences* (2012), 109(23), pp. 9179–9184.

10. Gilad, R, Hochner, H, Savitsky, B, Porat, S & Hochner-Celnikier, D., 'Castor oil for induction of labor in post-date pregnancies: A randomized controlled trial', *Women and Birth*, pp. 1–6. 2017.

11. Al-Kuran, O., Al-Mehaisen, L., Bawadi, H., Beitawi, S., Amarin, Z., 'The effect of late pregnancy consumption of date fruit on labour and delivery', *Journal of Obstetrics and Gynaecology* (2011), 31(1), pp. 29-31.

12. Kordi, M., Meybodi, F.A., Tara, F., Memati, M., Shakeri, M.T., 'The effect of late pregnancy consumption of date fruit on cervical ripening in nulliparous women', *Journal of Midwifery & Reproductive Health* (2014), 2(3), pp. 150-156.

13. Kordi, M., Meybodi, F.A., Tara, F., Fakari, F.R., Memati, M., Shakeri, M., 'Effect of dates in late pregnancy on the duration of labor in nulliparous women', *Iranian Journal of Nursing and Midwifery Research* (2017), 22(5), pp. 383-387.

14. Khadem, N., Sharaphy, A., Latifnejad, R., Hammond, N., Ibrahimzadeh, S., 'Comparing the efficacy of dates and oxytocin in the management of postpartum hemorrhage', *Shiraz E-Medical Journal* (2007), 8(2), pp. 64-71.

15. Dove, D & Johnson, P 1999, 'Oral evening primrose oil', *American College of Nurse-Midwives*, vol. 44, no. 3, pp. 320–324.

16. Smith, C.A., 'Homoeopathy for induction of labour', *Cochrane Database of Systematic Reviews* (2003), Issue 4. Art. No.: CD003399. DOI: 10.1002/14651858.CD003399.

17. Nishi, D., Shirakawa, M.N., Ota, E., Hanada, N., Mori, R., 'Hypnosis for induction of labour', *Cochrane Database of Systematic Reviews* (2014), Issue 8. Art. No.: CD010852. DOI: 10.1002/14651858. CD010852.pub2.

18. Holst, L., Haavik, S., Nordeng, H., 'Raspberry leaf – should it be recommended to pregnant women?', *Complementary Therapies in Clinical Practice* (2009), 15(4), pp. 204– 208.

19. Kavanagh, J., Kelly, A.J., Thomas, J., 'Sexual intercourse for cervical ripening and induction of labour' *Cochrane Database of Systematic Reviews* (2001), Issue 2. Art. No.: CD003093. DOI: 10.1002/14651858.CD003093.

20. Bovbjerg, M.L., Evenson, K.R., Bradley, C., Thorp, J.M., 'What started your labor? Responses from mothers in the third pregnancy, infection, and nutrition study', *The Journal of Perinatal Education* (2014), 23(3), pp. 155–164.

Chapter 8

1. Reed, R., 'Supporting women's instinctive pushing behaviour during birth', *The Practising Midwife* (2015), 18(6), pp. 13-15.

2. Brancato, R.M., Church, S., Stone, P.W., 'A meta-analysis of passive descent versus immediate pushing in nulliparous women with epidural analgesia in the second stage of labor', *JOGNN* (2008), 37(1), pp. 4-12.

3. Shorten, A., Donsante, J., Shorten, B., 'Birth position, accoucheur, and perineal outcomes: informing women about choices for vaginal birth', *Birth* (2002), 29(1), pp. 18-27.

4. Soltani, H., Hutchon, D.R., Poulose, T.A., 'Timing of prophylactic uterotonics for the third stage of labour after vaginal birth', *Cochrane Database of Systematic Reviews* (2010), Issue 8. Art. No.: CD006173. DOI: 10.1002/14651858.CD006173.pub2.

5. Mercer, J.S., Erikson-Owens, D.A., 'Is it time to rethink cord management when resuscitation is needed?', *Journal of Midwifery & Women's Health* (2014), 59(6), pp. 635-644.

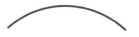

Index

Available from Pinter & Martin
*in the **Why it Matters** series*

Series editor: Susan Last

pinterandmartin.com